Prakruti

प्रकृति

Prakruti

Your Ayurvedic Constitution

by

Dr. Robert E. Svoboda

GEOCOM

Albuquerque, New Mexico
1989

This is a reference work.
It is not meant for diagnosis or treatment
and it is not a substitute for consultation
with a duly-licensed health care professional.

The exact transliteration from Sanskrit of the word *prakruti* is
prakrti. But, because Westerners have difficulty in pronouncing
it, it is usually written *prakriti*. However, spelling it *prakruti*
makes it easier to pronounce correctly, and is also in line with
the usage established by Dr. Vasant Lad in his books. Whenever
you elsewhere see the words *prakrti* and *prakriti*, though, please
remember that they are identical with *prakruti*.

First published in the United States of America by
Geocom Limited

© 1988,1989 Robert E. Svoboda
All rights reserved

ISBN 0-945669-00-3

Distributed to the trade by
Lotus Light Publications
P.O. Box 2
Wilmot, WI 53192
(414) 862-2395

Dedication

This book is dedicated to my parents, who were my first teachers, and to Vimalananda, who was my friend, philosopher and guide.

It is also dedicated to Mother Tara, the Universal Mother Nature from whom we all originate, in whom we all exist, and to whom we all eventually return. She is the Mother of compassion, forgiveness, truth, beauty, knowledge, abundance, energy, and freedom: She is equally well the Mother of darkness and bondage. From Her are born both sickness and health.

Motherliness is essential to healing, because Mother Nature alone can heal. This book is humbly offered to Mother Tara with the request that She heal all of us, and heal our world.

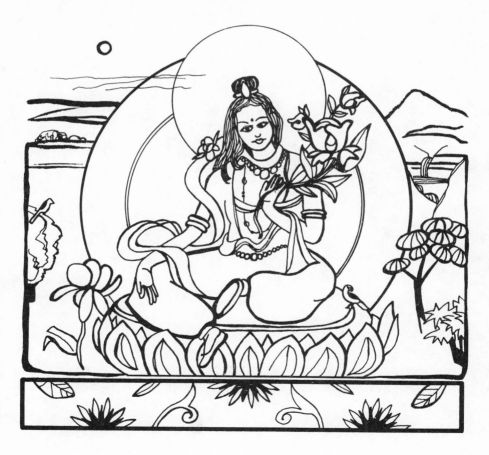

Foreword

Ayurveda encompasses not only science but religion and philosophy as well. We use the word religion to denote beliefs and disciplines conducive to states of being in which the doors of perception open to all aspects of life. In Ayurveda the whole of life's journey is considered to be sacred. The word philosophy refers to love of truth, and in Ayurveda, Truth is Being, Pure Existence. The source of all life, Ayurveda, is a science of Truth as it is expressed in life.

Ayurveda believes that every individual is a unique phenomenon. The individual is indivisible from the cosmos. Whatever is there in the macrocosm, the same thing exists in the microcosm. Every individual is a manifestation of cosmic consciousness.

The vibration of pure universal consciousness produces the soundless sound "Om." From this sound the five basic elements are produced, i.e. Ether, Air, Fire, Water, and Earth. Furthermore, these five basic elements are manifested into the three biological organizations known as Vata, Pitta, and Kapha. In every organism these three govern all physio-pathological changes.

At the time of fertilization, Vata, Pitta and Kapha determine by their permutations and combinations the constitution of an individual, which is called "prakruti." The "prakruti" means "the first creation." Every human being is the first creation of the cosmos, and that is why every human being is a separate entity, a unique phenomenon. To understand this uniqueness of every individual is the study of "prakruti;" Ayurveda gives us a direct approach to this study.

The healing science of Ayurveda is based totally upon the knowledge of "prakruti," the individual constitution. If every individual knows his own constitution, then one can understand, for instance, what is a good diet and style of life for oneself. One man's food is another man's poison. Therefore, to make one's life healthy, happy and balanced, the knowledge of constitution is absolutely necessary.

My friend and colleague Dr. Robert Svoboda studied Ayurveda at the Tilak Ayurveda Medical College in Poona, India. There, he was a student of mine whose understanding and brilliance in Ayurveda resulted in his standing first in his class. This achievement is more noteworthy because Dr. Svoboda is an American who is the only Westerner to have ever completed the program in an Ayurvedic Medical School. His profound knowledge of Ayurveda and his background in English combine to make this important work of his invaluable to the Western reader.

Dr. Vasant Lad, October 1987

Acknowledgements

The author would like to thank the following people who read and critiqued this book, or otherwise offered assistance for its generation:

Judy P. Allyn
Tyagi Kersten
Graham Dodd
Elliot McLaughlin
Vaidya B. P. Nanal
Fred & Kathy Smith
Laura & Edwin Svoboda
Vimalananda

Launette Rieb
Pamela Barinoff
Dr. Michael Stone
Dr. Vasant D. Lad
Michael Laurenson
Dr. Greg Heil (Krsna Das)
Loretta Levitz & David Liberty

Original art work by Donna Fish.

Table of Contents

Introduction

Nature and Her ways are truly inscrutable to mortals. You can set out on your life's journey intent on heading west, but if She wills you to go east your road will wind around until you are pointing eastward. When I left the U.S.A. on the Ides of March, 1973, I never suspected that I would end up living in India. I was enrolled in the University of Oklahoma Medical School, and expected only a brief African sojourn before returning to begin the September term.

A month later, however, I was lying on my back in Abidjan, Ivory Coast, violently ill with dysentery. Two Frenchmen had taken pity on me and had brought me back to their apartment to spend the weekend until I could locate a doctor. They were themselves on their way to what they described as a "witch doctors' convention," a gathering of healers, magicians, and trance mediums in the deep bush. Their guide was himself a "witch doctor." When he arrived and saw me lying inert on the bed, utterly exhausted, he insisted on treating me. I was too weak to object.

He was a well-dressed young African of thirty-odd years, with a robust physique. He could easily have been mistaken for a bank clerk, and had I had enough energy to think I would have thought that he was a most unusual witch doctor. But I was too weak to think, so I thought nothing of it when he poured a glass of water from the carafe near my head and began to stare intently into it. I watched him passively as he mumbled some sort of incantation over the glass and handed it to me to drink. I drank it passively, assuring myself that mere water could do me no harm even if it did me no good. The doctor and the Frenchmen bade me adieu, and I sank into a profound sleep.

When I woke I expected to feel the urgency of the disease, but was pleasantly surprised to discover that my abdomen was calm. It remained calm all that day and the next, and would have continued to remain calm had I known then what I know now about the effect of diet on disease. But the lesson was well taken: I had been temporarily cured by a shaman, with very little effort of faith on my part. During my next few days of convalescence in that flat I also read my first book on Yoga. Thus began the process which culminated in my move to India.

The next step occurred in Kenya where I participated with a team from the National Museum of Kenya on an ethnological expedition to the lands of the Pokot tribe. I was invited to join the tribe ritually, and did so. I met tribal medicine men and women, and chatted with

European M.D.s who testified to the usefulness of some of the tribe's traditional cures. I determined to study Pokot medicine more thoroughly, and promised myself to return to Kenya after a visit to Nepal.

In Nepal, however, the Peace Corps physician introduced me to the word Ayurveda, and the Tibetan Kalachakra initiation which I attended later in India introduced me to the practical benefits of Yoga. In spite of the misgivings I had from my first impressions of India I knew I had to remain there and study its ancient physical, mental, and spiritual healing arts.

The Art of Medicine

One of the first things I learned was that medicine is an art. Until then I had held the prevalent mechanistic view of life, that the human is basically a thinking machine and that disease and health are basically engineering problems. Ayurveda taught me that, like other arts, therapy becomes healing only when there is a healer involved. Artisans can paint pictures, craft pots, or compose concerti, but their products are lifeless unless, as an artist, they can breathe life into a creation. I know now that good medicine is the offspring of the marriage of art and science.

Cooking is a science, but no scientifically cooked souffle can compare with that prepared by a master chef. The chef may know nothing of the thermodynamics of food preparation, but he knows how to make his food delight the human palate. A master chef is an artist of cuisine. An Ayurvedic physician must be a good cook as well as a doctor, because good medicine is prepared just like good food. Cooking is one facet of Ayurvedic art, and Ayurvedic therapy succeeds only when the physician has as much a feel for the therapy as an expert cook has for an apple pie. Attunement to Nature provides this feel, and allows a doctor to approach the ideal of physician as intuitive healer. Ayurveda is not unscientific; it has progressed beyond science.

No doctor since the beginning of time has ever cured a patient. No doctor ever will, for Nature alone can cure. Physicians are not meant to work wonders or perform miracles. A true physician is a teacher who helps his or her patients work through their problems at all levels. Doctors are meant to use their knowledge of the patient's past illnesses and present conditions to intuit future possibilities for health and establish a healing strategy for the individual. True physicians leave the miracles to Nature, offering themselves as channels through which Nature can work Her magic. Every physician has the immutable obligation to exert maximum energy for cure at all times to all patients, even during diagnostic procedures.

More than a medical system, Ayurveda is a way of life, a way of cooperating with Nature and living in harmony with Her. Health in Ayurveda means harmony, and there is really no end to the degree of harmony you can achieve if you set yourself to the task. This method of living emphasizes prevention over cure, without neglecting cure. Some complain that Ayurveda works slowly, but slowness is often part of the remedy, especially today when many of us suffer from the disease of haste. Ayurveda balances and rejuvenates an organism, reducing its susceptibility and empowering its immunity to prevent new disease from developing.

We humans have not really changed much in our recorded history. Our technology is more advanced, surely, but our bodies and minds are almost identical to those of our ancestors, who suffered from the same diseases and demonstrated the same admirable and despicable qualities that we do. Ayurveda's unbroken chain of experience has much to say to us today. Its therapies, and its methods for determining the appropriate therapy for each condition, have been tested by thousands and thousands of physicians on millions and millions of patients. Its theories have stood the test of time.

In ancient days, when Ayurveda was being developed, humans were much less able to control their external environment than we can today. They had no choice but to rely on Nature. Lacking fancy instruments they cultivated their intuitive abilities, and because they lived in close proximity to Nature they found it easy to determine the medicinal effects of plants, animals and minerals. They experimented on themselves, and handed down their observations to their children. This collected medical lore was codified long ago in the form of Ayurveda.

The ancients used the human mind for their computer systems. They developed their powers of memorization so that each physician was a storehouse of copious medical fact, and they used their well-developed and refined powers of intuition to direct the therapy. They made Ayurveda into a healing art, and determined that the proper goal for a medical system should be no less than the achievement of immortality.

Health, Individuality, and Immortality

All humans have at one time or another dreamed of becoming immortal. Despite our knowledge that everything which is created is eventually destroyed, each of us secretly cherishes the hope that Death might in our one case make an exception. India's ancient Rishis (or Seers) studied this question and addressed it in their hymns, collected in the oldest compositions of the human race, the Vedas, which are the foundation of Indian culture. The Vedas emphasize that spiritual, mental and physical perfection are all equally essential for immortality. One famous Vedic prayer states:

Lead me from darkness into light.

Lead me from untruth into truth.

Lead me from mortality into immortality.

Because every embodied individual is composed of a body, a mind and a spirit, the ancient Rishis of India who developed the Science of Life organized their wisdom into three bodies of knowledge: Ayurveda, which deals mainly with the physical body; Yoga, which deals mainly with the spirit; and Tantra, which is mainly concerned with the mind. The philosophy of all three is identical; their manifestations differ because of their differing emphases. Ayurveda is most concerned with the physical basis of life, concentrating on its harmony to induce harmony of mind and spirit. Yoga controls body and mind to enable them to harmonize with spirit, and Tantra seeks to use the mind to balance the demands of body and spirit.

Yoga and Tantra are paths to freedom from dependence on the world. True freedom is the ability to be totally adaptable. Yoga relies on progressive restriction of inputs from outside; Tantra relies on transmutation of all external inputs so that one is no longer dependent on them, but can take them or leave them at will. Yoga and Tantra help make an individual independent.

Ayurveda was designed by the Rishis especially for those individuals who want to enjoy the world healthily. Its daily and seasonal routines, dietary guidance, therapeutics and doctrine of antidotes for the side-effects of addictions can keep you hale, hearty and having a high time well into your senescence if you can restrict yourself sufficiently to follow these precepts strictly. You must consciously choose how much you wish to indulge, which determines how healthy you will be. There is no free lunch.

Yoga traditionally encourages people to keep the world at arm's length, to live ascetically in order to limit the introduction of external disturbances into the internal environment. This approach works well but is too severe for most modern people. Tantra seems to provide unlimited indulgence under the cover of spirituality, but in fact true Tantra is an exceedingly rigorous system which can be successfully begun only after strenuous Ayurvedic purification and Yogic practices. Yogic and Tantric practices should not be followed without at least a rudimentary foundation of Ayurvedic knowledge.

Individual balance or harmony has a vertical dimension which is the dynamic interplay of the individual's body, mind and spirit; it's horizontal dimension is the equilibrium between the individual and his or her environment. Your physical body must be in balance with Nature, your mind must be in harmony with the group-mind of the society or group you live in, and your soul must be in a satisfying relationship with the Universal Soul if you are to be truly healthy. The Rishis used all life as their textbook; physicians must do the same, learning for themselves when and how it is appropriate to deal with a patient's body, mind, or spirit.

It is easiest to harmonize the body-mind-spirit complex by starting with the body, which is relatively stable. Balance of the mind and spirit, which are ethereal and therefore inherently difficult to stabilize, comes more easily once the body has been made firm and healthy. This is especially important today when most people are thoroughly enthralled with the material world. A physician must treat a patient at the level of consciousness on which the patient can respond, and since most people are submerged in physical consciousness, physical medicine should be first employed. Occasion to use mental and spiritual medicine inevitably follows.

Every human being is a unique individual, full of idiosyncrasies and peculiarities. Your most precious possession, your life, is yours and yours alone, unlike that of any other human being past, present or future. Each human is a unique manifestation of Mother Nature, the Creative Energy of the universe. Each possesses an indwelling fragment of the Universal Soul. The message of the Vedas is that each of us must find our own path to a life lived to the fullest, for only by making the most of ourselves can we repay to Nature the debt we owe Her for giving us life. The universe needs you to add your mite to the vast collective tapestry we call human civilization. You can make your fullest contribution to life only if you are healthy, and health alone enables you to enjoy your life to the fullest in return.

The word *Svastha* means "healthy" in Sanskrit. It is derived from:

Sva "self" + Stha "established" =

Svastha "established in the self."

The "self" here is the ego; not the Freudian ego, but the power of individual identity which separates every being from every other being. The ego is that which gives me my identity, which makes me know that I am I, not you, he, she, we, or they. The aspect of the personality which perpetually reminds me that I am I is called in Sanskrit *Ahamkara*, literally, "the I-former." Because each of us is a body, a mind, and a spirit, we each have a body-I, a mind-I, and a spirit-I. To be "established in self" is to be established in each of these selves.

Today's physicians tend to ignore individuality. They often look at people as "livers" or "lungs," and neglect the organism which hosts that liver or lung. Some espouse the therapy they know best as a cure-all for all the ailing, overlooking the variations which exist even among patients of the same illness. Such piecemeal therapy cannot encourage balance in the organism. Since today's doctors often fail to project health onto their patients, today's patients must learn to project health themselves. Everyone in today's world who wants to be healthy has a personal responsibility to learn as much as possible about health.

We all exist as individuals against the background of our external environment, Mother Nature. None of us can ever be wholly individual, because we are generated out of Nature, who conditions our individuality. Most of us embrace the world, indulging ourselves unlimitedly, relying on the world to continue supplying goodies to us and on Nature to provide us enough digestive power to consume them. Most of us call this self-indulgence freedom.

Enjoyment is certainly one of life's purposes, but you lose your ability to enjoy if your exceed your limits. Limitation is inherent in life. You are limited by dozens of obligations, such as the necessity to breathe, to eat, to sleep, and to use words to communicate with others. Your most important limitation is your organism's capacity to endure your indulgences.

Either you can willingly limit yourself or Nature will limit you. Disease is Nature's way of forcing you to slow down and rest. This is why She is called Mother Nature: She loves you so much that She cannot bear to see you ruining yourself. She warns you of your errors over and over, and turns to drastic measures only when you obstinately refuse to listen to Her. It is a classic case of freedom versus responsibility: either you restrict your freedom a little bit each day, or Nature will come along and restrict it for you for days, weeks, or months at a time.

Indulgence is a legitimate life goal, but it is only one of four life goals. No life is completely lived unless each of these goals is achieved. They are:

Dharma, the goal of fulfilling the duties assigned to us by our positions in society;

Artha, the goal of accumulating possessions in the course of fulfilling our duties;

Kama, the goal of satisfying legitimate desires with the assistance of one's accumulated possessions; and

Moksha, the goal of realizing that there is more to life than duty, possessions and desires.

You need a stable niche in society in order to arrange for the necessities of life and the leisure to permit you to live either a life of indulgence or one of spiritual asceticism. Whatever your life aim, you need a sound mind in a sound body to achieve it. You have to be healthy if you want to enjoy yourself continuously.

Many Westerners will study Ayurveda in hopes of finding miracles which will allow them to continue going about their self-indulgent ways.

They may find temporary relief, but permanent relief comes only with permanent changes in lifestyle. These people cheat themselves as much as people who flock after miracle-mongers in hope of effortless spiritual advancement. Ayurveda is for those who are ready to take responsibility for themselves.

If Ayurveda were a religion, Nature would be its Goddess, and over-indulgence would be the sole sin She would punish. Ayurveda is meant to allow you to enjoy the pleasures of life up to the point that such enjoyment interferes with your health. Full-time gratification is in fact bondage, because the more we consume the more we become captives of our consumption. Unlimited indulgence makes us less free because we become less self-sufficient. Each of our addictions—to caffeine, sugar, salt, sports spectaculars, TV game shows, alcohol, drugs, gambling palaces, or other indulgences—is another nail in the coffin of our freedom, another restraint to individuality. Most of us don't even know how to indulge properly, and we sicken and die from the side effects of our indulgences. True enjoyment is possible only where there is true health.

I have been travelling around the USA, talking to people about Ayurveda and trying to find out what Ayurveda can do for them. This book is one result of my travels. It is not an exposition of the classical principles of Ayurveda; in fact, an old-line Ayurvedic physician might well take issue with me over some points. It is my own interpretation of certain Ayurvedic theories. I am indebted to my teacher Vimalananda for these observations, for he taught me to think in this way.

Darshana, the Sanskrit word for "philosophy," literally means "seeing." Philosophy is therefore words which allow you to see things in a certain way. Ayurveda is a philosophy which allows physicians to see patients the way Nature sees them. The sages who created Ayurveda were called "Seers" because of their ability to perceive reality clearly. They could see how the world and its parts operate, and could describe their observations in words which allowed those who would come later to see and perceive in the same way. Each Seer saw things from a different viewpoint, so there are many systems of Ayurveda, not just one. Following this tradition, every Ayurvedic physician has his or her own individual system, derived from the experiences of the Great Seers and augmented by personal experience. This book is a partial exposition of my own experience.

It begins with an introduction to fundamentals of the Ayurvedic world view and shows how these principles determine constitutional types. Then it proceeds to consider the effects of food on constitution, the inner nature of nutrition, and good habits for establishing and preserving health.

The subject matter then strays into topics which explore the forces which bind body, mind and spirit together, concentrating on Ahamkara and the nature of individual identity. Because you are healthy, or Svastha, when you are established in your self, it is important to examine how this establishment in self comes about and is maintained, and how it is affected by addiction. There is an examination of disease causation, using obesity and arthritis as two examples of the Ayurvedic approach to disease management. Finally reproduction and rejuvenation in the light of Ahamkara are used to introduce more esoteric methods of self-balance.

Many Sanskrit tomes open with the word "atha," which means "now," indicating that the book's knowledge is waiting within, ready to be experienced at any time by whoever opens it. Ayurvedic knowledge is perennial and universal, as valid today as it was 5,000 years ago and as it will be 5,000 years from now. Details may change, specifics may come and go, but the essence of the knowledge remains inviolate. I have studied the ancient Ayurvedic writers, like Charaka, Sushruta and Vagbhata, both in translation and in the original Sanskrit. Taking their teachings to heart, I have tried to apply the essence of their ancient wisdom to the specifics of our modern problems. Ayurveda is quite complex; I have taken the liberty of removing from it a few teachings which I feel can act as initial tools for those of us who want to improve ourselves.

One major modern problem is rootlessness, a disease which is promoted by the great mobility of today's people. We Americans pride ourselves on the fluidity of our culture, which is the world's melting pot. Ours is a society in which everyone can, theoretically, use talent and ambition to earn fame and fortune. Every man a king, at least of himself, is our motto. We revel in our rootlessness, and love to live footloose, free of all ties and limitations of the past. Most of our ancestors came from other countries to forget their pasts. Forgetting the past became an American rite of passage. In magnifying our individuality thus, we came to equate progress with forgetfulness, and now Progress, as epitomized by Science, has become our idol. Most of us continue in our way, slaves to Progress.

Allegiance to progress makes us tend to confuse individuality with sovereignty. A strong sense of individual identity is important to the health of all humans beings, but in older societies in which all members shared a culture, an individual was not solely responsible for defining his or her identity. A Japanese, for example, knows that he or she is an inheritor of the ancient culture of Japan. Much of his or her personality develops from adoption or rejection of the tenets of that culture, such as reverence for parents, elders, and Emperor.

America's cultural institutions are much less deeply ingrained in us, and Americans are in general much less willing to respect the past than are other peoples. Since we have less past experience for soil in which to plant the seeds of our personalities, we must rely more on our own individual experience. Each of us establishes an individual ethic and morality. This is the culmination of egotism. Unfortunately, most of us invest a lot in our individualities, since we have nothing else to invest in with confidence. We have a collective policy of *sauve qui peut* (everyone for oneself) which regards everything outside the individual, even Nature, as an enemy.

Forgetfulness is a devastating disorder. We modern humans have forgotten our roots, we have forgotten our gods, and we are now busily trying to forget our morals. We feel freer and less constrained the more we forget, unaware that each additional loss of memory distances us further from our true identities. We construct for ourselves false personalities derived from the veneer of addictions to our sensory indulgences, defining freedom as unlimited gratification, forgetting that all individuality is conditional. Cut off from communication with our internal mother we are severed from our source of compassion, and we forget how to empathize with other living creatures.

This is why many of us do not hesitate to eliminate anything which is either not part of us or has no demonstrable benefit to us. Thus our society is violent. Our literature, our art, our music, even our agriculture is violent, and our medicine is equally violent. We kill with antibiotics and antiseptics, and if our slaughter is ineffectual we use surgery to expel the offending organ from our presence. We destroy the body in order to save it.

"Establishment in the self," however, does not mean cutting yourself off from your source, the being Who has created you. Overinvestment in self is as unhealthy as its opposite. Destruction should be a last resort; nurturance, a motherly feeling of nurture and support for oneself and for all beings, should be the first resort. Nature is always magnanimous, and She will be as generous to you as you are generous to yourself and to other beings. You cannot buy, beg, borrow or steal health; it is Nature's gift to you.

Ayurveda is the product of a civilization which is deeply rooted in Mother Nature. The Seers knew that all of Nature is part of the individual, since we all are created from, exist in, and return to Nature. Individuality is therefore a very temporary condition which can flourish only with the assistance, not the enmity, of Nature, the permanent condition.

Carl Jung expressed this opinion after a visit to India in 1938:

"It is quite possible that India is the real world, and that the white man lives in a madhouse of abstractions…. Life in India has not yet withdrawn into the capsule of the head. It is still the whole body that lives. No wonder the European feels dreamlike; the complete life of India is something of which he merely dreams.

When you walk with naked feet, how can you ever forget the earth?"

This book is meant to reintroduce Westerners to "walking with naked feet" through life, to come back into contact with Nature. Although centuries old, the concept of individual constitution is a new concept for the Western mind, a new way for all of us to understand our "relationship" with Nature. Ayurveda is above all meant for all people who by harmonizing themselves seek to act as harmonizing forces in the universe.

Our overweening, arrogant passion for self-indulgence has poisoned our world. If we hope to continue living on this planet, we must now reverse the damage, both in ourselves and in our environment, so that we can calm Nature's ire and return ourselves to health. The purpose of the Science of Life, as Vimalananda often said, is to make every home a happy home, a home in the true sense of the word: a haven. Everyone should have a real home, a haven they can always go home to, inside and outside themselves. All of us have a Mother in Nature, and only She can lead us home.

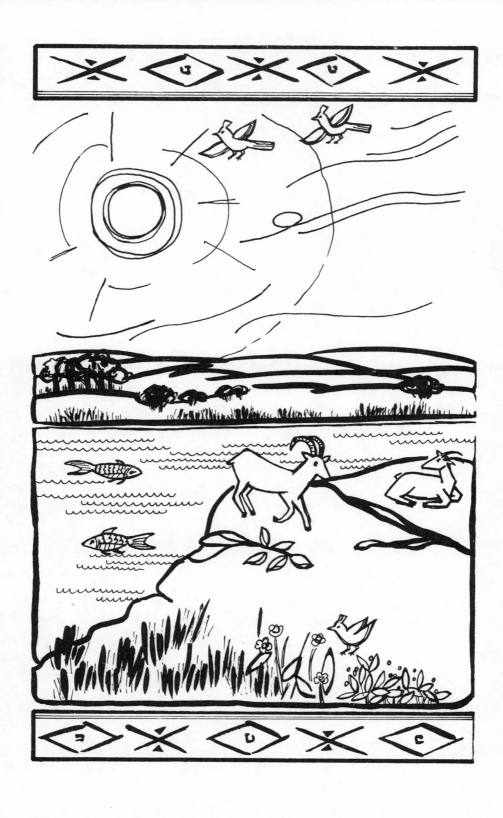

Chapter One
Doshas and Tastes

Each of us maintains separateness from other living beings for as long as Nature permits us to remain alive. Nature gives us the space bounded by the skin and the digestive tract to call our own. Every thing outside the skin is part of the environment. You are a part of my environment, and I am a part of your environment. Nature is the sum total of all individuals and their environments.

Inside your digestive tract is material which was originally part of your environment. Once it had its own separate existence, its own individuality; now it is on metabolic probation, attempting to pass the digestive exams to become a part of you. Should your gastro-intestinal tract rupture, some of this material will escape into your body cavity. Because your body can recognize it as alien a tremendous reaction will occur, which if allowed to progress will kill you very quickly.

Should your external skin fail to do its job, as might occur after severe burns, alien marauders will enter your system, which may also result in your demise. We owe our continued day-to-day existence to the admirable fortitude of our twin boundaries, the external skin of the body and the internal skin of the gut.

Diseases are beings with parasitical intentions. Some have collective bodies, like worms, bacteria and viruses, and show signs of collective consciousness just as social insects like ants and termites do. Other diseases have no bodies of their own and "take possession" of an organism in order to express the compulsions of the individual existences. Still others, entities like cancer, are created within the body. Whatever the intruder, cure occurs when the alien personality is expelled from the organism and the host's innate personality returns to normal.

Aliens are unwelcome in a healthy body. An unbalanced system encourages improper digestion of food, which produces physical and mental toxins, called "Ama" in Sanskrit. Ama acts as food for parasites, and encourages them to thrive in the organism. Indigestion develops because of poor eating and living habits, deliberate, willful indulgence in unhealthy practices which are collectively called "Prajnaparadha," or "crimes against wisdom." Indigestion prevents nutrients from reaching the tissues, and weakens the host's immune defenses.

The aura is the first line of defense against parasitical beings. The second line of defense is formed by the skin and the gut. A third line of defense, the immune system, awaits to intercept and destroy any parasites which somehow find their way past the first two defenses. The immune system, which communicates with both the skin and the gut, is a sense organ, a "sixth sense" for intruders. It is an intricate web of T-cells, B-cells, antibodies and lymphokines, a system of fascinating complexity all controlled by a single boss: Ahamkara.

Ahamkara ceaselessly identifies itself with each of the trillions of cells in the body. Your Ahamkara constantly reminds every one of your cells of its identity as a sub-unit of that grand and glorious entity known as You. The Ahamkara ensures that only those cells which swear allegiance to its overlordship are allowed to remain alive in the body. All aliens are hunted down and ruthlessly slaughtered, and all rebels—mutant or cancerous cells—are mercilessly executed as a warning to other cells who might dare to resist your rule.

You can remain alive, safe inside your castle, only so long as your Ahamkara serves as your garrison governor. When she is injured, alien beings may find a weak spot in your defenses and strike you down. When she, the warder who forces your cells to slave away for you, relinquishes her charge, all the inmates are free to go their own ways, and you die. She is your wife, your lover, your friend, your guide and advisor, and your servant. She is your all-in-all. Above all, she is your mother.

Ahamkara is feminine because she is a fraction of the Divine Mother Goddess Nature. She is your wife because she is always with you, bonded in the marriage of body to mind to soul which is you. She is your lover because only the power of her love can bind all your cells together and induce them to function in concert as a unified being. She is your friend because she is always there to sympathize with you. She guides and advises you regarding your self-interest. As servant, she tirelessly slaves away to keep you running.

Most important of all these aspects is her relationship to you as mother. The "I am" principle aggregates to itself all the building blocks which form you: the Five Great Elements which create the body, the sense organs, and the mind. You are born because of the "I-former," so she is your mother. The ancient Rishis knew this well, and worshipped their own Ahamkaras as mothers in order to enter into loving relationships with them. India is a motherland because the Rishis in their transcendent wisdom recognized the creative importance of Mother Nature. Even Adi Shankaracharya himself, the originator of ten sects of renunciate monks who shun all normal human interactions, mandated worship of the Goddess in all his monasteries.

Diseases arise when Ahamkara is afflicted and immunity weakens. The Sanskrit word for immunity is Vyadhikshamatva, which translates literally as "forgiveness of disease." You retain your health only so long as you are willing to forgive your stresses, shrug off adversity and adapt to new situations. Resistance to change always impedes the workings of the immunity. An old Sanskrit proverb tells us, "Kshama cha janani": the essence of motherly love is forgiveness. Damage to the Ahamkara-mother weakens our innate forgiveness and predisposes us to disease.

Treatment of Ahamkara is the ultimate medicine. India's sages have long known that good spiritual health is a prerequisite for good physical and mental health. Spiritual health is a dynamic balance between a strongly integrated individual personality and the cosmic personality of Nature, a balance which is possible only so long as a being remembers its debt to Mother Nature.

Only immortal beings can be completely healthy, because only they have so empowered their own Ahamkaras that no alien being can ever invade them. India's ancient Rishis performed long penances to completely awaken and control their Ahamkaras, and they became immortal in consequence. Because they wanted to communicate their experiences to others, they established the system of philosophical "seeing" which students of Ayurveda use to look at embodied life.

When the wise Rishis examined their own experience and consulted their intuitions they realized that human consciousness, will and identity must be fragments of Nature's own consciousness, will and identity. The subtlety of their faculties of perception allowed them to contact Nature and communicate with Her directly. One of the first things they learned concerned the structure and origin of the universe.

Nature told them that first exists

Pure Existence

which experiences desire for manifestation,
and splits into

Consciousness and *Will*

which then mate together. Their offspring is

Intellect

which is the power of discrimination.
Intellect then evolves into

Ahamkara

Which is the "I-former." The universe fills with numberless little bundles of intellect with individuality, all searching for a means of expression. According to their innate predilections these Ahamkara-bundles manifest as:

waves of kinetic energy, *Rajas*

material particles of potential energy, *Tamas*

and subjective consciousness, *Sattva*

Rajas is activity, Tamas inertia, and Sattva the balance of both of these; consciousness alone can balance kinetic energy with potential energy. Nature's Ahamkara is sufficiently vast to balance the energies of the entire cosmos. The I-consciousness in humans is sufficient to balance their own individual energies.

An individual bundle of "spirit," desirous of expressing itself, uses subjective consciousness, or Sattva, to manifest sense organs and a mind. Spirit and mind then project themselves into a physical body, created from the Five Great Elements which arise from Tamas. The sense organs use Rajas to project from the body into the external world to experience their objects. The body is the mind's vehicle, its instrument for sense gratification. The mind retreats to its bodily haven each night during sleep when it is tired of roaming about outside. The spirit remains within this haven at all times, providing life to the body and consciousness to the mind.

The Five Great Elements

Just as our bodies are made up of trillions of independent cells, we are all little cells in the universal organism. Like our cells, each of us humans has an individual existence but none of us is "free" enough to live independently of the whole. In fact, everything which exists in the external universe has its counterpart in a living being's own personal internal universe. Every cosmic force is represented, in altered form. The flow of nutrients into and wastes out of body cells also characterizes the continuous flow of nutrients and wastes into and out of plants, animals and humans.

There is therefore no inherent difference between, say, cooking your food in a pot on the stove and cooking your food in the pot of your stomach on the stove of your internal digestive "fire." Both use heat to prepare the food for easier assimilation. Flames are used on the external stove and acid and enzymes on the inside, but the principle of cooking is identical to both.

The Rishis used the theory of the Five Great Elements, more properly known as the Five Great States of Material Existence, to explain how the internal and external forces are linked together. The Five Great Elements are:

Earth the *solid state* of matter, whose characteristic attribute is stability, fixity or rigidity. Earth is stable substance.

Water the *liquid state* of matter, whose characteristic attribute is flux. Water is substance without stability.

Fire the power which can *convert a substance from solid to liquid to gas*, and vice versa, increasing or decreasing the relative order in the substance. Fire's characteristic attribute is transformation. Fire is form without substance.

Air the *gaseous state* of matter, whose characteristic attribute is mobility or dynamism. Air is existence without form.

Ether the *field* from which everything is manifested and into which everything returns; the space in which events occur. Ether has no physical existence; it exists only as distances which separate matter.

The Three Doshas

These Five Elements condense to the Three Doshas: Vata, Pitta and Kapha, which are effectively Air, Fire and Water respectively. Vata is the principle of kinetic energy in the body. It is mainly concerned with the nervous system, and controls all body movement. Kapha is the principle of potential energy, which controls body stability and lubrication. The tissues and wastes of the body which Vata moves around are Kapha's province. Pitta controls the body's balance of kinetic and potential energies. All of Pitta's processes involve digestion or "cooking," even if it is the cooking of thoughts into theories in the mind. The enzymatic and endocrine systems are Pitta's main field of activity.

At the cellular level Vata moves nutrients into and wastes out of cells, Pitta digests nutrients to provide energy for cellular function, and the cell's structure is governed by Kapha. In the digestive tract Vata chews and swallows the food, Pitta digests it, Vata assimilates nutrients and expels wastes, and Kapha controls the secretions which lubricate and protect the digestive organs. In the mind Vata retrieves previous data from memory for comparison with new data. Pitta processes the new data and draws conclusions, which Vata then stores as new memories. Kapha provides the stability needed for the mind to grasp a single thought at a time.

These three are forces, not substances. Kapha is not mucus; it is the force which when projected into the body causes mucus to arise. Pitta is not bile; it is the force which causes bile to be produced. Vata is not gas, but increased Vata causes increased gas. Vata, Pitta and Kapha are called Doshas because the word Doshas means "things which can go out of whack." When Vata, Pitta and Kapha are out of balance with one another the system is bound to lose its own balance.

Kapha, the Watery Dosha, is actually associated with both the Water and Earth Elements, which have no real affinity for one another. When you pour sand into water, for example, it drops to the bottom of the vessel and sits there. No matter how hard you try the sand will remain suspended in the water only so long as you continue to stir. Although some solid substances like common salt dissolve in water, most others do not. Kapha is that force which Nature has provided to us to keep the body's Earth (its solids) suspended in its Water (its liquids) in the proper proportion.

Wherever the body becomes too solid a problem always develops. For example, gall stones and kidney stones. These are concretions of Earth in which Water has dried out too much to permit free flow to continue. Likewise, when there is too much Water and not enough Earth in the system, disturbances like edema can result. Kapha forces Water and Earth, which would otherwise refuse to interact with one another, to combine properly and remain in balance.

Pitta, the Fiery Element, is associated with both Fire and Water. While Water and Earth would love to be able to ignore one another and are inert to each other when they do mix, Fire and Water are always antagonistic. Whenever you mix Fire and Water together, one or the other is bound to come out uppermost. If there is more Fire than Water, Fire boils off or evaporates Water; if there is more Water than Fire, Water even when boiling hot drowns out Fire. To make two such opponents cooperate together is Pitta's job.

All "fires" in the body are contained in water. Stomach acid, for example, is an extremely powerful acid, with a pH of 2. It burns anything it touches, just as an open flame or a bolt of lightning burns. Acid is Fire contained in Water. When Fire predominates in this mixture, the acid burns through the natural containment facilities which Water provides. If this happens in the stomach, a gastric ulcer results. When Water predominates it douses the Fire, creating indigestion. Only the mediation which healthy Pitta provides can keep this uneasy alliance of Fire and Water intact.

Air and Ether compose Vata. Air, like wind in the external universe, can move freely in the body only when its path is free of obstacles. You are safe from strong wind in your home, unless the wind happens to be so strong that it blows down your walls. Likewise, insufficient empty space (Ether) prevents proper movement of Air, unless Air's force accumulates sufficiently to blast a free passage for itself.

Ether is totally inert; Air is totally mobile. Air always attempts to expand itself free from limitations. If this tendency becomes too pronounced all limiting structures are destroyed. Excessive empty space and insufficient power of movement can also result in stasis, with adverse implications for health. Emphysema is an example of such a condition; another is the type of constipation that develops after overuse of enemas or colonics. Only healthy Vata can keep Air and Ether balanced with one another. Vata's task is to ensure that there is just sufficient Ether for Air to move in.

These three Doshas have qualities, or attributes, which characterize their effects on the organism. They are :

Vata	Pitta	Kapha
dry	oily	oily
cold	*hot*	cold
light	light	*heavy*
irregular	intense	stable
mobile	fluid	viscous
rarefied	malodorous	dense
rough	liquid	smooth

Vata possesses all the qualities we usually associate with air. It dries, just as even a mild, moist breeze eventually dries clothes hung on a line. It cools, just as even a hot wind can cool a body by evaporating sweat from its skin. It roughens, just as the desert wind erodes the mesas and buttes of the desert. It is erratic, or irregular; it usually comes in puffs and gusts, not as a steady stream. Wind is not rough in itself, nor need it be dry or cold to cause dryness or coldness. Its innate qualities take precedence over the conditional qualities it picks up from its environment.

Pitta likewise produces its effects because of its own innate characteristics. It is oily, or unctuous, not because fire is oily but because oils and fats burn brightly in fire. Like fire it is hot, intense, and light, and its fluidity and liquidity derive from the fact that it is Fire contained in Water. Because it is fluid and can engulf and devour food it is able to digest and transform.

Kapha has all the same qualities as mucus. It is viscid, which makes it slow-moving. It is also cold, heavy, dull, thick, smooth, sticky, and sluggish, all qualities which we associate with mud, a substance composed of Earth suspended in Water. Yogurt is a characteristic example of a Kapha-type food because it too possesses all these attributes.

Note that:

Both Pitta and Kapha are oily, and Vata is dry, so *dryness* is characteristic of Vata. Dryness appears in the body or mind only when there is disturbance of Vata.

Dryness is a side-effect of *motion*, which is Vata's physiological function. The *unevenness* of excessive dryness introduces *irregularity* into the body and mind.

Both Vata and Kapha are cold, and Pitta is hot, so *heat* is characteristic of Pitta. Heat appears in the body or mind only when there is disturbance of Pitta.

Heat is a side-effect of *transformation*, which is Pitta's physiological function. The *intensity* of excessive heat introduces *irritability* into the body and mind.

Both Vata and Pitta are light, and Kapha is heavy, so *heaviness* is characteristic of Kapha. Heaviness appears in the body or mind only when there is disturbance of Kapha.

Heaviness is a side-effect of *stability*, which is Kapha's physiological function. The *viscosity* of excessive heaviness introduces *slowness* into the body and mind.

Because Vata, Pitta and Kapha all possess their own unique inherent qualities, they have distinctive affinities for certain bodily organs. They are all present in each cell, since they are essential to life, but they tend to congregate in certain areas:

Vata	Pitta	Kapha
Brain	Skin	Brain
Heart	Eyes	Joints
Colon	Liver	Mouth
Bones	Brain	Lymph
Lungs	Blood	Stomach
Bladder	Spleen	Pleural Cavity
Bone Marrow	Endocrine	Pericardial Cabity
Nervous System	Small Intestine	

Vata and Kapha are almost totally opposite one another in quality. Kapha, which represents all potential states of energy in the body, permits energy to be stored. Vata, which represents all kinetic states of energy in the body, causes stored energy to be released. Vata promotes change, but excessive change can lead to overstimulation. Kapha promotes stasis, but excessive stasis can lead to inertia. Pitta is in charge of balancing these two diametrically-opposed forces.

Vata and Kapha congregate near one another for practical reasons. The heart and lungs are continuously in motion and so require continuous lubrication. Vata provides the motion, Kapha the lubrication. Too much motion uses up the lubricant; too much lubricant gums up the works. In the joints, synovial fluid provides lubrication and protection. The brain and spinal cord, whose movement is confined to nerve impulses, swim in cerebrospinal fluid. Mucus protects the lining of the gut throughout its length, enabling the food within it to pass freely. Movement and stability, and the force which balances them: Vata, Kapha, and Pitta.

Vata, Pitta and Kapha are all essential to life, but can cause great harm if they are allowed to fall out of harmony with one another. This two-faced personality exists because they are Doshas, things which are often in error. This is not really their fault, because they have such difficult jobs to do. Kapha must overcome the mutual indifference of Water and Earth and make them work together, Pitta must conquer the natural animosity which Water and Fire feel for one another, and Vata is forced to use the inert Ether to try to control the capricious Air. It is in fact surprising that they function as well as they do.

Because they are so reactive the body cannot afford to store them within itself for long, any more than a nuclear power plant can afford to store radioactive wastes. They are therefore eliminated from the body regularly in the course of performing their functions. The force of Kapha is continually expelled from the body via mucus, Pitta is regularly excreted through acid and bile, and Vata is eliminated both as gas and as muscular or nervous energy.

The Six Tastes

Regular elimination of the Doshas is important because normal metabolic processes continuously produce them. How much of each Dosha your body produces depends primarily on which Tastes you consume. The Tastes influence the balance of the Doshas in the body. Like the Doshas they are derived from the Five Great Elements. They are capitalized here to emphasize the profound effect they have on all parts of the organism, not merely the tongue:

Sweet - Composed mainly of Earth and Water, Sweet increases Kapha, decreases Pitta and Vata, and is cooling, heavy, and unctuous. It nourishes and exhilarates the body and mind, and relieves hunger and thirst. It increases all tissues.

Sour - Composed mainly of Earth and Fire, Sour increases Kapha and Pitta, decreases Vata, and is heating, heavy, and unctuous. Sour refreshes the being, encourages elimination of wastes, lessens spasms and tremors, and improves appetite and digestion.

Salty - Composed mainly of Water and Fire, Salty increases Kapha and Pitta, decreases Vata, and is heavy, heating, and unctuous. Salty eliminates wastes and cleanses the body, and increases the digestive capacity and appetite. It softens and loosens the tissues.

Pungent - Composed mainly of Fire and Air, Pungent (which is hot and spicy like chili peppers) increases Pitta and Vata, decreases Kapha, and is heating, light, and dry. Pungent flushes all types of secretions from the body, and reduces all Kapha-like tissues such as semen, milk and fat. It improves the appetite.

Bitter - Composed mainly of Air and Ether, Bitter increases Vata, decreases Pitta and Kapha, and is cooling, light, and dry. Bitter purifies and dries all secretions, is anti-aphrodisiac, and tones the organism by returning all Tastes to normal balance. It increases appetite, and controls skin diseases and fevers.

Astringent - Composed mainly of Air and Earth, Astringent (which makes your mouth pucker) increases Vata, decreases Pitta and Kapha, and is cooling, light, and dry. Astringent heals, purifies, and constricts all parts of the body. It reduces all secretions, and is anti-aphrodisiac.

All these Tastes are essential for proper functioning of the organism, and reach us primarily through our food. My teacher Vimalananda always maintained that it's not what you eat, it's what you digest that counts. The healthiest food in the world is the deadliest of poisons if you cannot digest and assimilate it properly. Digestion begins in the mouth at the instant the tongue Tastes the food. The food's Tastes are transmitted directly to the brain, which determines what sort of fat, protein or carbohydrate has been ingested and what sort of juices need to be secreted for optimal digestion. By the time the food reaches the gut, the digestive organs must be ready for it.

Diners who praise delicious dishes misdirect their praise, because Taste is really present in the mouth, not in the food. A food which is described as Sweet, for example, is a food which is experienced as Sweet by most healthy individuals under ordinary conditions. Normally an orange Tastes both Sweet and Sour, but according to the condition of your sense of Taste you may sometimes Taste it as Sweeter and sometimes as more Sour.

As an experiment, cut an orange into two halves and eat one half. Then take a teaspoonful of something Sweet, like honey or maple syrup, and finally eat the other half of the orange. No matter how Sweet the first half seemed, the orange's second half will Taste less Sweet, more Sour. Your organ of Taste, not the orange, has changed. The Sweetener you took temporarily satiated your body's capacity for Sweet. When the second half of the orange entered your mouth, your tongue ignored the Taste it had plenty of and selectively experienced Sour, the orange's other Taste.

Another example of the internal nature of Taste utilizes a leaf from India, Madhuvinashini, which translates as "Killer of Sweet." It temporarily abolishes the Sweet Taste when chewed. Even after a small quantity, sugar loses its Sweetness, and your tongue experiences only its texture rather than its Taste. Since sugar's sole Taste is Sweet, it becomes just like soluble sand. Apples retain their Sourness even after the Sweet is gone; licorice root loses its Sweetness and retains most of its Bitterness. Some Bitterness is lost because this leaf also reduces Bitter slightly. Sweet and Bitter are two sides of the same coin.

Taste does not disappear from food even after it is digested. Each of your cells has a rudimentary sense of Taste, and each is affected by the Taste of its nutrients. Since each cell in your body affects every other cell, and since all those cells affect your senses and your mind, the Tastes in the food you eat exert a critical influence on your consciousness and your health. Taste predominates over all other physical influences on the individual, even the Doshas, because Taste is the first input from ingested food that the system receives.

Everything you eat has three opportunities to affect your organism:

The effect a food has on you *before digestion* begins is the taste your tongue picks up from it while it is in the mouth. This effect is called *Rasa*, or *Taste*.

The second effect, which is experienced *during digestion*, is the food's *Virya*, or *Energy*. "Hot" food increases the body's ability to digest, freeing energy for other metabolic tasks. "Cold" food requires extra energy for its digestion. The gut obtains this energy from the rest of the body, which must reduce its other activities as a result.

The *Vipaka*, or *Post-Digestive Effect* is that which occurs after digestion is over and the nutrients are assimilated deep within the tissues. Sweet and Salty usually produce a Sweet, satisfying, nutritive effect after being digested, a net gain for your organism. Sour usually produces a Sour effect, increasing the desire for new things to digest but neither adding to or subtracting from yourself. Bitter, Pungent and Astringent generally produce Pungent, which causes things, physical and mental, to be consumed or to flow out of you. Bitter and Astringent reduce Pitta because even though their Post-Digestive Effect is usually Pungent (which increases Pitta) because their cold Taste and Energy more than compensate for the Pungency produced.

Taste	Energy	Post-Digestive
Sweet	Cold	Sweet
Sour	Hot	Sour
Salty	Hot	Sweet
Pungent	Hot	Pungent
Bitter	Cold	Pungent
Astringent	Cold	Pungent

Sour, Salty and Pungent are always "hot," and Sweet, Bitter, and Astringent are always "cold," but sometimes it happens that a substance may have a heating Taste with Cold Energy, which means that when it enters the body it increases the digestive power but during digestion it does not aggravate Pitta. Sometimes it may be the other way round: a substance may have a cooling Taste and Hot Energy, reducing appetite when it is eaten but increasing digestive juice flow while digestion is going on.

For example, cooked onions are Sweet in Taste, Hot in Energy, and Sweet in Post-Digestive Effect. They satisfy hunger with their Sweet

Taste and promote anabolism with their Sweet Post-Digestive Effect, but their Hot Energy does not permit Kapha to be disturbed by their Sweetness.

Lemons are Sour and Bitter in Taste, Cold in Energy, and Sweet in Post-Digestive Effect. Being Bitter they tone the body and prevent Kapha increase; being Sour, they increase digestion and appetite and relieve Vata. Their Cold Energy prevents Pitta from being disturbed, and their Sweet Post-Digestive Effect means they assist in tissue nutrition. The substances which most effectively balance the organism are usually those which are most unique in their pattern of qualities.

EFFECTS OF OVERUSE

You can maintain balance among the Six Tastes as long as you do not persist in overusing one or more of them. The effects of overuse of specific Tastes include:

Sweet - obesity, diabetes, dropsy, parasites, obstructed circulation, eye inflammation, indigestion, vomiting, gas, lethargy, respiratory congestion, and other Kapha-type disturbances.

Sour - burning sensations, itches, giddiness, premature aging, looseness of body, suppuration.

Salty - inflammation, edema, easy bleeding, skin diseases including herpes and hives, joint disease, impotence, early wrinkling of the skin, early baldness.

Pungent - pain, dizziness, loss of consciousness, dryness of the mouth, tremors, debility, emaciation, burning sensations, fever, increased thirst, drying of sexual secretions.

Bitter - all Vata diseases including numbness, emaciation, cutting or breaking or colicky pain, giddiness, headache, stiffness, tremors, decreased sexual secretions.

Astringent - all types of Vata disturbance including tremors, fits, constipation, dryness of the body, distention, tingling numbness, emaciation, thirst, decreased sexual secretions.

Salty is the most important Taste for control of Vata, because it is heavy, oily and heating, and improves digestion. Sour comes next, and then Sweet. Bitter is the best Taste for control of Pitta, because it is cooling and drying. Sweet comes next, and then Astringent. Pungent is the best Taste for control of Kapha, because it is heating, light and dry and flushes secretions from the body. Bitter comes next, and then Astringent. The intensity of the Tastes in a food determines its effects on the Doshas.

Two of the first physical manifestations of disturbance in body tissues are the mistaking of one Taste for another, and the inability to experience Taste at all. Both these disturbances usually result from overuse of one or more Tastes. This dullness of the Taste sense makes it impossible for the brain to properly prepare the body for the incoming food. This prevents proper digestion.

The Six Tastes are even more important to the mind than they are to the body, because of the mind's craving for sensory stimulation. There are two groups of senses: the five senses of perception, which we all know well, and the five senses of action, which are the voice, hands, feet, genitals, and anus. Each sense of perception is a channel through which the mind moves to a sense object, experiences it, and returns to process its experience. Each sense of action is a channel into which the mind enters in order to express itself by projecting its personality into the outside world, and through which it returns again after completing its expression.

Like any other channel, the sensory channels can suffer from disease: they can either be too dilated or too constricted. Overuse of a sense organ overdilates its channel, enervating that sense so that the mind can no longer obtain any enjoyment from its use. Underuse of a sense constricts that sense organ's channel which also reduces the mind's ability to enjoy itself along that pathway. An overdilated channel provides too much Ether for Air to move properly in; an overconstricted channel is an obstruction to Air's unimpeded movement. Overuse, underuse, misuse and abuse of the sense organs are collectively regarded in Ayurveda as one of the three main causes of human disease.

PREDOMINANT EMOTIONS

Of the many factors which influence the dilation and constriction of the sensory channels, the most important are probably Taste and emotion. The Sanskrit word Rasa means, among other things, both "taste" and "emotion." According to the conventions of Sanskrit grammar, this suggests that Taste and emotion are identical forces on different planes of existence. In fact, Taste is to the body what emotion is to the mind. An emotion in the mind tends to produce in the body its corresponding Taste, just as ingestion of a specific Taste tends to create in the mind its corresponding emotion. The predominant attitudes and emotions associated with the Tastes are:

Sweet - satisfaction, or satiation (the "sweet taste of success"). Overindulgence in Sweet leads to its negative aspects, complacency and greed.

Sour - the searching outside oneself for things to possess. Sour causes evaluation of a thing in order to determine its desirability which selectively enhances certain appetites. Overindulgence in evaluation leads to envy or jealousy, which may manifest as deprecation of the thing desired, as in the "sour grapes" syndrome.

Salty - zest for life, which enhances all appetites. Overindulgence in zest leads to hedonism, the craving for indulgence in all sensory pleasures physically available to the body, just as an "old salt" or a "salty dog" will do when he enters port again after a long sea voyage.

Pungent - extroversion, the tendency to excitement and stimulation, and particulary the craving for intensity. Overexcitement and over-stimulation lead to irritability, impatience and anger ("pungent language," or "a sharp retort").

Bitter - dissatisfaction, which produces a desire to change. When you have to swallow a "bitter pill," its bitterness dispels your self-delusion and forces you to face reality. Too much disappointment leads to frustration, which confirms your system in bitterness. Grief is also Bitter.

Astringent - introversion, the tendency away from excitement and stimulation. Excessive introversion leads to insecurity, anxiety and fear. Astringency causes contraction, which makes you "shrivel like a prune," and clamps the "cold, bony hand of fear" around your throat.

At all times your personality tries to maintain itself in the greatest possible comfort. It seeks the satisfaction of Sweet, and will make use of any other Taste it requires to obtain it, selecting "hot" or "cold" Tastes according to its requirements. Sour, Salty and Pungent are "hot" Tastes and Sweet, Bitter and Astringent are "cold" Tastes. Each of their corresponding emotions is accordingly hot or cold. Heat expands and cold contracts; this is a universal principle of physics. Cold constricts physical and mental channels; heat dilates them.

Sweet, Bitter and Astringent are cooling Tastes, and their corresponding emotions are cold and contracting. They decrease the organism's desire to "eat" new things. Satisfaction or complacency is a constricting emotion because it lessens the mind's appetite for enjoyment through a sense. Dissatisfaction constricts because it is an admission of inability to enjoy through a sense. Fear constricts all senses; it is the most powerful of all constricting emotions. Fear actually produces constriction in the bronchioles of susceptible individuals and can initiate asthmatic attacks.

Sour, Salty and Pungent are hot Tastes, and their corresponding emotions are hot and expansive. They increase the organism's desire to consume food or other sense objects. This is hedonism, Salty's emotion. Envy or jealousy actively increases the mind's desire to enjoy, Anger indirectly increases the physical and mental appetites by flooding the organism with heat.

Salty is called "all-tastes" Sarva Rasa in Sanskrit because it can enhance all flavors in a food while simultaneously increasing the organism's appetite for food. It promotes good digestion when used in small amounts as a condiment, but weakens the body when used in excess. "Hedonism," the emotion associated with Salty, does the same for the mind: small amounts increase the mind's desire for intensity of experience, but overuse makes the mind vapid and weak.

Salty forces the body to retain water, and increases the production of digestive juices and sexual fluids, which is why salt is contraindicated in those who wish to remain celibate. In fact, Salty increases all body juices. Life itself is based in water—each of us is 75% water—so more juices make for a "juicier" life as your senses, powerfully impelled by Salty to gratify themselves, force you to immerse yourself in worldly pursuits. Salt and the Salty Taste are intoxicants, literally, and like all other intoxicants possess a potential for abuse.

EFFECTS ON CONSCIOUSNESS

Actually, all Tastes can be used as intoxicants. Sweet, for example, is a popular drug in our society. People use it to make themselves feel satisfied. Some societies intoxicate themselves with the envy of Sour or the irritability of Pungent, and some individuals may even use Bitter and Astringent for self-gratification. We all use our food to alter our consciousness, and all alterations of consciousness affect the body via the Three Doshas:

Sweet's - intense complacent effect increases the naturally inert, complacent Kapha, cools the anger of Pitta and comforts the fear of Vata.

Sour's - envious effect increases Kapha if envy of another's success incites you to obtain further success for yourself. Otherwise Pitta will increase as jealousy mutates into anger over the raw deal you feel you are getting from life. Envy does help reduce Vata, by focusing and heating up your consciousness.

Salty's - "hedonism" increases complacency as long as you are able to indulge, which increases Kapha. It increases the fieriness of Pitta's anger whenever there is any obstruction to your gratification, and decreases Vata by allaying fears of inadequacy or inability to properly indulge.

Pungent - increases Pitta by actively increasing the flow of hormones and digestive juices, making it easier both to digest and to manifest anger. It relieves Kapha by decreasing self-satisfaction, and temporarily relieves Vata by permitting expression of bottled-up resentment. In the long run, however, Pungent increases Vata by exhausting the organs and glands, which "dries you out," limiting your ability to project aggression or unhappiness outwards.

Bitter - is the best of all Six Tastes. As Dr. Vasant Lad says, "Bitter is better." In small amounts Bitter helps balance all other tastes in the body. Just as mild dissatisfaction with yourself or your situation impels you to change, Bitter dilates channels which are too constricted, thus reducing Kapha and its complacency, and constricts those which are overdilated, thus reducing Pitta and its anger. Overuse of Bitter, though, increases Vata, as dissatisfaction and continuous change induce insecurity and fear.

Astringent - constricts, drawing one away from the self-satisfaction of Kapha and the self-aggrandizement of Pitta. Its constriction increases fear of insufficient sensory "nutrition" and leads to increased Vata.

Bitter, Pungent and Astringent all increase Vata and decrease Kapha. Their lightness reduces your desire to remain connected with your body, and makes it more difficult for your personality to self-identify with your body even if it wants to continue to do so. Sweet, Sour and Salty all increase Kapha and decrease Vata. Their heaviness enhances both your ability to self-identify with your body and your interest in doing so. We are all prey to our Tastes and emotions.

For example, we live in a consumer culture. In order for our economy to continue to function we are all expected to go deeply into debt. To promote spending, Madison Avenue through its advertising wizardry creates new desires within us for things we never before had and usually do not need. First the desire for a hedonistic lifestyle is created, which creates the Salty Taste within us. Next comes envy, as we compare ourselves to the Joneses next door and realize how much more and better they are able to gratify their senses than are we. This produces the Sour Taste. Finally, our impatience to be able to gratify ourselves manifests as anger when some obstacle comes in our way; this creates Pungent.

Salty, Sour, and Pungent, the Hot Tastes. We are now "all heated up," ready to consume and digest, physically and mentally. All remains well as long as we are able to obtain enough "food" (for any of our senses) to satisfy this hunger. Inevitably, however, some of these created desires remain unfulfilled. Even with unlimited wealth at your disposal, there are a limited number of hours in the day. How much can you spend? How much can you gratify yourself? The desires which remain unfulfilled create Bitterness within you because of your dissatisfaction.

Ayurveda teaches us that in small doses Bitter is a tonic for the appetite and digestion. It works this way in the world as well; a little dissatisfaction spurs you on to greater and greater appetites. Too much dissatisfaction though, creates an excess of Bitterness in the organism. When you don't have sufficient energy—money—to go around, you have to prioritize your indulgences, and this leads to frustration because repeated, constant enjoyment is projected at you ceaselessly in the media. Excessive Bitterness overstimulates Vata and disturbs your mind as you brood over your state.

Sour, Salty, and Pungent perfuse your being while you have the interest and ability to indulge, and once your indulgence is interrupted Bitter floods your organism. Your body knows it has a Taste imbalance, and knows that Sweet can be used to rebalance the situation, so it craves Sweet. Sweet satisfies the hungers generated by Sour, Salty and Pungent, and being Bitter's exact opposite it eliminates frustration and dissatisfaction. Once Sweet is consumed the body and mind temporarily return to balance and feel pleased with themselves.

The mind does not have to consume food in order to obtain Sweetness. It can derive Sweet from any thrill-producing activity, even a shopping spree. The temporary sensation of unlimited power inherent in a credit card provides powerful gratification, which unfortunately disappears almost as soon as the purchaser returns home with the purchases.

Well-digested food satisfies longer than other thrills can because, even after the initial rush of pleasure is gone, properly digested and assimilated food will be nourishing and gratifying thousands of body cells. Unsatisfactory digestion creates the same secondary dissatisfaction that results from any other cheap thrill, flattering only to deceive. The tissues are momentarily taken in by the promise of substantial nutrition, and feel jilted when the smoke clears and the sensation is gone.

Even when there is good digestion, the intensity of the Sweet sensation abates as soon as the food has been digested and assimilated. The tendency then is to eat again, to experience again the temporary somatic bliss which food affords. This tendency is even more pronounced if digestion is poor, because despite food intake little nutrition actually reaches the tissues, which then send messages to the mind to remind it that they are starving. The more you eat in such a condition, the weaker your digestion becomes.

Soon the individual begins to crave Sour, Salty and Pungent as well as Sweet because the "hot" Tastes enkindle the digestive fires to permit further gratification by food. Sour, Salty, and Pungent also enhance the appetite, however, so no matter how much you eat you will always be hungry for more.

Fast food, which now accounts for half of all meals served in the U.S.A., developed because no one knows when a craving for immediate gratification of the tongue may arise. Think of French fries: the potatoes are themselves Sweet, and they are served with a thick frosting of Salt, and slathered in Sweet-Sour-Salty ketchup. The eater gets his or her Sweet fix with sufficient Sour and Salty to awaken the taste buds and the digestive organs. Or the noble hamburger: Sweet-Sour mayonnaise plus Sour-Salty-Pungent mustard plus Sweet-Sour-Salty pickles all on a Sweet wheaten bun. And the taco, which has all these Tastes plus an increased quantity of Pungent to further stimulate an already overstimulated digestive tract.

Junk "foods," which are junk because they are all taste and no nutrition, are usually washed down with soft drinks or coffee. Most soft drinks are intensely Sweet, and many have the added bonus of caffeine. Coffee is Pungent, plus whatever Sweet is added with cream and sugar, and is also full of caffeine. Caffeine is a metabolic credit card, a substance which forces the body to secrete enough hormones to keep us functioning, gratifying ourselves with Sweetness in its various forms until we drop from fatigue. Like the fiscal debt we are encouraged to create, most of us develop crushing burdens of physiological debt by use of such "credit cards."

Eventually all the bills come due. Unlike Third World countries, your organism cannot default on its debts, except by dying. Perhaps diabetes develops, a disease in which the body can no longer cope with the tremendous quantities of Sweet which the mind requires, and begins to discard it undigested. Or maybe your thyroid or adrenals collapse from their debt burden and your system goes on a general strike.

Your personal constitution, which is your individual metabolic makeup, helps determine how much effect specific tastes and emotions have on you. This is why everyone who eats the same food does not necessarily suffer from exactly the same mental or physical effects from it. When all the members of a family enjoy a meal together, each individual's tastes and emotions will be affected according to his or her own individual taste and emotional balance.

Your inborn metabolic pattern is called "prakruti." Prakruti also means Nature, She who is the first creation. Your prakruti is your first "creation," your first reaction when you are forced to adapt to some change in your environment. Your constitution is that set of metabolic tendencies which determine how your body and mind will instinctively react when they are confronted by a stimulus. Many of the traits you prize in your personality arise from and are dependent on these metabolic tendencies. Many of the qualities you dislike in yourself also arise from these tendencies. Knowing your constitution allows you to know your body and mind better. You learn why there is no need to feel guilty for your dietary preferences, or for your mental traits like anger or fear. Once you understand that these traits are determined by your constitution, lifestyle changes can help your organism minimize their influence.

Your personal constitution was determined by the state of the bodies of your mother and father at the time of your conception. That certain sperm which could best endure the conditions prevalent in those two bodies won the race to reach the ovum, and its genes mingled with the genes in the ovum to form the new child. Your constitution is influenced by your parents' genetics, by your mother's diet and habits during her pregnancy, and by any abnormal events at the time of your birth. Once your personal constitution and its accompanying tendencies have been set they cannot be permanently altered. Like your genes, you have your constitution for the rest of your life, like it or not.

You can, however, learn to adjust for your constitution so that you are less affected by its distortions. You can learn how to prevent health imbalances and how to best treat them when they arise. You can know the prognosis of any disease you might contract, and you can determine which rejuvenation program will be best for you. Through study and use of Ayurvedic principles you can also understand why your spouse, children, relatives, friends, neighbors and co-workers do the things they do, and determine how best to interact with them for maximum inter-personal harmony. You can plan meals for your family according to what is best for each of their prakrutis.

Ayurveda is a very common-sense sort of medical system. It uses very simple, easy-to-understand principles to determine individual prak-ruti. These principles are based in the theory of the Three Doshas, and therefore your prakruti is expressed in terms of Vata, Pitta and Kapha. Vata-type people actually are more Airy and Ethereal than are other people. Their bodies tend to produce more intestinal gas, and their minds tend to be more "spacey." Even the crackling noise their joints make is said by some authorities to be due to the displacement of bubbles of nitrogen in those joints. Pitta-type people literally have more Fire in them than do other types. They have better appetites and better diges-tion, can withstand cold better, and are more hot-headed. Kapha people tend to have heavier, earthier bodies than do other types, and tend to store Watery substances like fluids and fat more readily than do others. Ayurveda looks at individuals through the lenses of Vata, Pitta and Kapha.

Your constitution also influences your emotions. For example, if you have a constitutional tendency to Vata increase you will be anxious and fearful by nature. You will naturally crave Sweet, Sour, and Salty, which reduce Vata and thus assuage fear. However, if you overeat Sweet, Sour, and Salty, trying to feel better and better, you will increase Kapha, which can obstruct the free movement of Vata and produce disease. To be healthy Vata people should eat mainly Sweet, Sour and Salty foods in amounts small enough to be easily digested.

People who are mainly Kapha constitutionally sometimes use Sweet, Sour and Salty to further entrench themselves in their set ways, when they should be using the Bitter, Pungent and Astringent Tastes to shake up and awaken themselves. It is not possible to stay alive on Bitter, Pun-gent and Astringent alone, but these Tastes should form a significant portion of the diet.

People who have Pitta-type constitutions are naturally aggressive and impatient. Sweet, Bitter and Astringent are the best tastes to combat this innate tendency and promote balance. Unfortunately Pitta-type people frequently choose Sour, Salty and Pungent food, which makes them even more aggressive, impatient and ruthless, and revs them up for greater and greater achievement, which is a hallmark of the Pitta personality. Such food tends to overheat their bodies and minds, however, and leads to imbalance.

Your constitution affects your emotions, and the Tastes you crave, via your genes. Scientists have already located a gene which produces depression when activated, and they are sure to find other genes which produce the other emotions which flesh is heir to. Each emotion may not be controlled by one single gene, but since all mental states have a physical basis there must be a gene or genes which produce a protein which interacts with a hormone which produces the emotion. And vice versa—your emotions can trigger certain of your genes to work and others to remain dormant, thus affecting your hormones and your metabolic balance.

If your parents and grandparents were easily angered, there is a strong likelihood that they will pass down to you a gene or a set of genes that will make you prone to anger easily. If they were fearful, they will probably pass a fear gene or genes down to you, and you will be dogged by fear all your life. Each of us lives in an emotional ocean spawned from these genes.

These genes are activated and deactivated by the Tastes we ingest, but they themselves never change; they always lie in wait for an opportunity to display themselves. As long as your genes exist, your tendency to certain emotions will stay with you. Until you can change your genes you will have to rely on knowing your own personal constitution if you hope to bring yourself into balance. Understanding your prakruti gives you insight into why you do the things you do, and can give you clues on how to improve yourself.

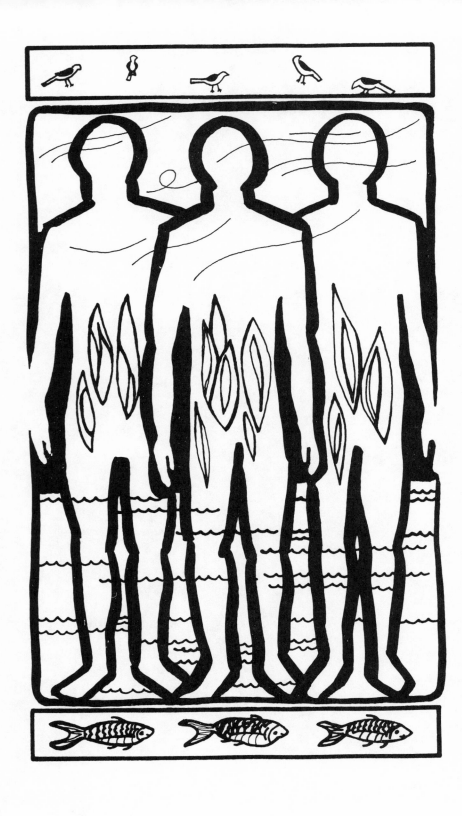

Chapter Two

Constitutional Characteristics

There are eight possible constitutional types:

V, P, K, VP, PK, VK, VPK, and Balanced.

The small number of VPK individuals who have all three energies imbalanced are rarely healthy and must live a very disciplined life to remain disease free. Also, the small number of individuals who are almost perfectly balanced are usually healthy since they must be severely stressed before an imbalance develops. We will concentrate on the other six types, the great majority of people. For convenience, Vata has been abbreviated to V, Pitta to P and Kapha to K.

To determine your own individual constitution, evaluate yourself as accurately and as honestly as you can. Avoid the temptation to see yourself as you would like to be rather than as you are. It is best to have a friend or family member evaluate you as well and then compare the two evaluations to ensure clarity. There is no right or wrong, and no better or worse, in this examination. There is only the reality of your personal constitution. Everyone passes who answers this exam honestly, and everyone fails who doctors their answers to make them conform more closely to their perceived self-image. Although you may not like your constitutional proclivities they are yours, and like mooching kinfolk they will stick with you as long as you live. You may as well learn to live with them, and learn how to change your life so you can be as healthy as you possibly can.

Please respond below according to how you have reacted in general throughout your entire lifetime, not how you react at present. Select the description which fits you most perfectly overall. If in any category there have been great changes at various times in your life, please select Vata as your answer even if the Vata description in that category does not accurately describe you as you are today. For example, if you have had wide fluctuations in your weight all during your life, so that you were significantly overweight at certain periods and almost underweight at others, you should answer "Vata" for your weight even if you are overweight at present.

Most people are not purely Vata or Pitta or Kapha in nature; most fit predominantly into one category and secondarily into another, because your constitution is derived from the conditions of the bodies of both your parents at the time of your conception. Unless they were both very close to one another in body type and health, the variation between them at that moment shows up as a variation in your constitution. If in any one category you feel that you belong partly in one constitution and partly in another, write down both. If in any one category you feel you might fit into all three constitutions select the two which best characterize you. Whenever there is significant doubt or confusion, select "Vata."

While evaluating yourself, keep in mind that:

Vata is *cold, dry* and *irregular.*

Pitta is *hot, oily,* and *irritable.*

Kapha is *cold, wet,* and *stable.*

Each constitutional type has its own inborn approach to the management of physical and mental energies which it applies to any variety of energy it encounters. Vata is governed by kinetic energy, the energy of action, and therefore V people make active use of their energy. They spend freely and frequently waste their energies because of this predilection for kinesis. K types are governed by the potential energy of Kapha and have a decided tendency to store energy within themselves. They have a genetic predisposition to save and steward energy well. Pitta is in charge of balancing and managing Vata and Kapha, and P people are born experts in managing and using efficiently energies of all sorts. Whether it be activity, money, speech, sex, or even sleeping and dreaming, an individual's innate pattern of energy utilization depends upon his or her prakruti.

Vata exerts a cold, dry, irregular influence on the system because as soon as energy enters the organism it is expended, leaving emptiness behind. Kapha has a cold, wet, stable influence and a K-type person is rarely empty because most of the energy which enters the individual remains stored within. Pitta's effect is hot, oily and irritable because Pitta must maintain a high level of reactivity in order to manipulate energy effectively.

Bear in mind that most people have a dual personality, and it will not always be easy to know which force predominates in you. If you feel confused, ignore the difficult categories and pay more attention to the easier ones. Narrow shoulders and/or hips almost always occur in V people; broad shoulders and/or hips are characteristic of Kapha. People whose skins are dark or who tan easily have a lot of Vata, while those who cannot tan at all or tan very little are very Pitta, especially if their hair is fine. The criteria listed for evaluation may seem complex because of the difficulty in describing in words concepts which are easy to see but hard to explain. Remember that Ayurveda is based in common sense, and rely on your own common sense to understand and use it. Each of the categories below will help illustrate to you the approach which your system follows in its own energy utilization.

Prakruti Evaluation

BODY FRAME

V people tend to be either unusually tall or unusually short. Because they grow like weeds, they are most often slender or rangy, with a thin body frame and narrow shoulders and/or hips. Frequently their arms or legs seem unusually short or, more often, unusually long. They tend to have long, tapering fingers and toes. Any significant departure from any body proportion is usually due to Vata's quality of *irregularity*.

V people may have very light, small bones, or heavy bones with joints which are prominent or protrude. Their joints often make cracking noises when they move. If you show most of these characteristics you are V, even if you are overweight. Most structural abnormalities, like deviated nasal septum, scoliosis, bow-legs, or knock-knees, are also due to Vata.

P people have medium frames with medium shoulders and hips, and normal joints. Their fingers and toes are medium in length. Their body frame and height are generally proportional and *balanced*, indicative of prudent use of energy for development.

K people have a medium to broad frame with a *heavy* bone structure and wide-set shoulders and/or hips. Their tendency to store energy encourages massiveness; football linemen are usually quite K in constitution. Their bodies seem well-proportioned to the eye, and their joints are well-lubricated, and may be deep-set. Their fingers and toes tend to be short and squarish.

WEIGHT

Vata's *dryness* promotes natural leanness of body. Some V people live out their lives in thinness and find it hard or impossible to gain weight, like my grandfather who could eat four meals a day and never gain an ounce. Such an individual's Vata expends all food energy which enters the body before it can be stored. V people are often skin and bones, with prominent tendons and veins on their limbs. Some Vs may overeat poor foods and become fat, but as they improve their habits and their diets and begin moderate exercise they can lose that weight and keep it off without much difficulty. V people are known for wide variations in weight even without radical changes in diet. They usually store most of their fat around their midriffs in a "spare tire."

Ps can usually maintain an average weight for their build, with minor fluctuations. They can usually gain and lose weight fairly easily, since Pitta is the body's principle of *balance*. They tend to deposit fat evenly all over their bodies.

K people can maintain moderate weight with regular exercise; otherwise Kapha's *heaviness* tends to make them add excess poundage. They gain weight easily, especially in the lower parts of the body such as the rear end, and lose weight with difficulty, since they innately enjoy having ample stored energy.

SKIN COLOR AND COMPLEXION

Your personal skin color depends greatly on your racial background. A Scandinavian who seems dark-skinned to his family will still be several shades lighter in pigment than the lightest African. Compare yourself with members of your immediate family or with others who have the same racial mix as you do to make an accurate evaluation.

Vs tend to be naturally dark, or they tan deeply and do not burn easily. They usually adore heat and cannot get enough sun, because they feel more "alive" after getting sun. Their bodies need regular infusions of heat because Vata is by nature *cold* since it does not store enough energy to maintain good bodily warmth. Because of innately poor circulation their skin is usually cold to the touch, and may have a grayish cast to it.

Ps have light-colored skin, often pink or coppery in hue. Because Pitta is *hot* and reactive their skin is usually warm to the touch. Their circulation is strong, but they tend to high blood pressure. They freckle before they tan, and rarely tan very deeply. They do burn easily, and may suffer from sun allergy.

K people enjoy the sun and burn after overexposure, but adjust easily to intake of solar energy and tan evenly and thoroughly after moderate sunbathing. Their skin is cool but not cold to the touch, but because they have good circulatory tone they rarely suffer from cold hands and feet as Vs often do. They may have a few freckles, but never in P-profusion.

SKIN CHARACTERISTICS

Vs tend to have problems with *dry* skin because their high energy output quickly uses up any available external lubrication. Their skin may be dry all over, or dry in patches and oily in patches due to Vata's quality of *variability*. V skin chaps easily and may have a leathery texture to it. It is susceptible to conditions like psoriasis and dry eczema. Corns and calluses form readily, as do cracks, especially on the bottoms of the feet. V types often suffer from chapped lips. They may have a few moles or wrinkles. Their body hair is either scanty or overabundant, and tends to be dark, coarse, and curly.

Ps usually have delicate, *irritable* skin prone to rashes and pimples, and inflammations like impetigo. They usually have many moles, and their skin tends to wrinkle early. The body hair is light-hued and fine-textured. Their skin is coppery-red in color, especially after exercise or when they are agitated. Their lips are deep red, reflecting the ample volume of blood beneath the skin. This also explains why Ps blush easily.

Ks have slightly oily, smooth, *thick* skin which is well lubricated, with a moderate amount of body hair and a mole or two. Ks are not naturally prone to any skin disorder. Their lips are full and moist.

SWEAT

V sweat is scanty even in heat because the V bodytype is metabolically *cold* and has a natural need for external heat sources like stoves, steambaths, and hot springs. V people who become overweight, however, perspire more.

Ps may sweat even in cold weather, because of Pitta's innately excessive *heat* production. Even P palms may seem sweaty.

K sweat is moderate, and is *consistent* even in climatic extremes.

HEAD HAIR

Hair is closely related to Prana, the body's vital force. This is the reason why like Samson none of India's Rishis ever cut their hair. They allowed it to grow as long as it liked and to break off when it chose to do so. Because healthy hair rarely grows on an unhealthy body, the hair and its luster are important indicators of overall tissue health.

V hair is usually *dry*, but may *vary* from dry to oily in different spots on the head. It is ordinarily dark in shade and is coarse or rough in texture. V hair is usually very curly or even frizzy, and tends to kink or tangle. It may be prone to dandruff or split ends, and often seems dull and lusterless.

Everyone with naturally red hair has substantial Pitta in their prakruti. Other Ps are those people with light-colored (blonde or light brown) hair, or those whose hair has gone grey or white at an early age. Early baldness is also a P-indicator, since it indicates high levels of testosterone, a hot, aggressive, P-type hormone. P hair is usually thin and fine or delicate, and quite straight. Sometimes oiliness dims its luster.

K hair is most characteristically brown or dark brown, or chocolatey, and is thick, slightly wavy and borders on coarseness. Oiliness is one of its chief disorders, but its luster is usually good.

NAILS

Vs have hard, brittle nails which are rough and may differ in size from one another. As always, significant *irregularity* shows a significant degree of V. Their nails often display marked ridges or depressions and may be slightly bluish or grayish in color. People who bite their nails as a habit are often V types.

P nails are soft, strong, somewhat rubbery, and well-formed. They are a lustrous pink in color, with a coppery tinge due to the profuseness of *warm* blood right under the skin.

K nails are strong, large and symmetrical, in line with Ks natural *regularity* and lack of variation. They tend to thickness and may seem somewhat pale in color.

EYES

Your eye color is that wavelength of light the body does not desire and so reflects back instead of absorbing. Grey eyes, for example, indicate that the body does not need grey, and since grey is one of the colors associated with Vata this demonstrates that a grey-eyed organism has ample Vata and needs no more.

Some people have brown patches in their eyes which indicate accumulated toxins in the system. These splotches do not represent the true eye color, though they may indicate a current condition. They should be ignored while determining constitution, and only the underlying color considered.

Eye size is subjective, but if your eyes seem small, just as an elephant's eyes seem small in relation to the size of its head, or if they appear unusually close together or far apart, they are V in nature. Grey, violet, and slate blue are the typical V eye colors. Very dark brown eyes, verging on the black of bittersweet chocolate, are also indicative of V. Individuals whose eyes differ in color from one another are usually V types. V eyes are often *dry* and scratchy. There is a grayish or bluish tinge to the sclera, and the eyes themselves quickly become dull and lusterless when the individual has expended all his or her energy and is out of sorts.

P eyes are medium in size and light in color. Hazel, green, red, light blue, and those electric blue eyes which some red-haired persons have are all P eye colors. P eyes usually burn with an intense *fire* and radiate energy in all directions. The sclera have a reddish tinge, and become fiery red when irritated.

K eyes are large and liquid, sometimes blue but more often milk chocolate in color. Their calm, cool, *stable* strength made the Ayurvedic texts compare them to the eyes of a deer or the petals of a lotus. They may have a tendency to itchiness.

MOUTH

V people tend to have crooked or uneven teeth, or buck teeth. Vata's *irregularity* may make the jaw too small to accommodate all the teeth, or too large for all the teeth to fit together snugly. Usually some teeth are significantly larger than others. V teeth tend to be brittle and oversensitive to sensations like cold and sweets. V gums often recede early. The tongue is often coated, and the coating is usually thin and adherent, and grayish or pinkish-grey in color. They may have an Astringent or Bitter Taste in their mouths when they wake up in the morning.

P mouths have even teeth of medium size. Their teeth are prone to cavities, and their gums tend to bleed easily. Their tongues are coated occasionally, and the coating is usually yellow, orange, or red. Sometimes the tongue is so *irritated* that it will bleed. The P mouth and tongue are also prone to canker sores. Ps may experience a Sour or metallic Taste in their mouths early in the morning.

Ks have large, even, gleaming teeth which rarely need attention. Their tongues are rarely coated, and when they are the coating is usually thick and curdy, and white, off-white, or greenish-white, associated with a sickly Sweetish Taste in the mouth.

APPETITE

V people are always anxious to eat, but their eyes are bigger than their stomachs; they feel full after eating less than they wanted to eat. Their appetites are *variable*: excessive hunger on one day may be followed by disinterest in food the next. People who become dizzy or faint unless they are assured of regular between-meal snacks are also Vs. They do not enjoy stringent fasting because their bodies do not store enough energy to carry them through long periods of food deprivation.

P people have good appetites and really enjoy eating. They are always ready to eat, morning, noon, night, and midnight, and hate to miss meals. Ps become snippy or *irritable* if they fail to eat when they are hungry, and they are not fond of fasting either because their systems are always on the prowl for new energy to consume and "manage."

K people have a *stable*, usually moderate desire for food, though they may be prone to emotional eating. They can go an entire day on water or juice alone without feeling any physical distress because they store plenty of energy in anticipation of such periods of deprivation.

BREAKFAST

Vs often find it difficult to function efficiently if they miss breakfast, because by mid-morning they begin to feel anxious or sleepy as their blood sugar drops and their energy becomes exhausted. Many Vs like a heavy breakfast, because they feel like they burn up their food quickly, but most feel better if they have a light breakfast and then an early lunch. Vs tend to rely on the caffeine in coffee or tea to wake them up and get them going in the morning, but this insidious practice robs them of energy later in the day, and eventually exhausts them altogether by *drying out* their glands. V energy comes in spurts or bursts anyway, and artificial stimulation by caffeine or sugar exhausts the energy reserves quickly.

P people can skip breakfast when necessary, especially if they are driving themselves toward some goal, but by lunchtime they begin to become *hot* and testy, and really calm down only after a good feed. Sometimes they suffer from heartburn when they are away from food for too long. They may take coffee and tea, but stimulants are less important to them in the morning to wake up than they may be during the course of the day to maintain their high levels of energy expenditure.

K people find they do best with a light breakfast, like a piece of fruit, and often enjoy skipping breakfast entirely. They usually are not much perturbed even if they miss lunch. They are not naturally attracted to stimulants, but may enjoy a cup of coffee or tea in the morning to help mobilize themselves.

DIGESTION AND EVACUATION

For the purposes of this question, anyone whose bowels do not regularly move once daily without straining or use of laxatives can be considered to be constipated. A condition in which loose stools are passed three or more times a day constitutes diarrhea. Healthy bowels move once or twice daily without assistance.

Some V people are lifelong sufferers from constipation, with a tendency to hard, dark-colored stools and frequent gas or bloating. Other V types experience *variations* in their bowel habits, with periods of constipation alternating with spells of loose stools or diarrhea. Many V people know from experience that good eating habits are essential for good digestion. When they are constipated, pure V people often respond only to strong laxatives like senna or castor oil.

P people are rarely constipated, and usually defecate regularly and frequently. Their stools are usually yellowish and well-formed, but sometimes are loose and may seem *hot* and burning, especially after a hot, spicy meal. An intense yellow or orange stool indicates great Pitta intensity in the body. Many P people find that substances like milk, figs, raisins or dates act as laxatives for them.

K people are usually *regular*, and move their bowels once daily. They are sometimes slow in their eliminations. Their stools are most often well-formed but are rarely hard. When constipated they respond to medium-strength laxatives.

MENSTRUATION

V women tend to have very *irregular* cycles, and may miss periods especially if they exercise too much or their weight drops too low. The spacing between periods is often longer than a month. Their flow tends to be scanty, and there may be clots. Both these symptoms are due to Vata's *dryness*. The blood is usually dark in color. Constipation and severe cramps may develop just before the bleeding begins. V cramps are generally more intense than are P or K cramps because cramping is itself due to Vata.

P women usually have regular cycles, but bleed for a longer time and more heavily than do others because of their innate *heat*. The blood is usually an intense, bright red. P women may have loose stools during or just before their periods, and may suffer from medium-strength cramps.

K women often have effortless, regular periods, with an average quantity of blood which may be rather light in color. Any cramps are likely to be mild, and are dull rather than intense. K women tend to be prone to water retention.

CLIMATE PREFERENCE

V-types are so *cold-blooded* that they love warmth at all times. It takes a lot of heat to make them sweat. The sun enlivens them, and they tend to lose strength during the dead of winter, when they bundle up warmly and seek out external sources of heat to make up for their meager internal heat production.

Pure P people prefer the colder latitudes and find hot climates intolerable. Because they produce so much internal *heat* themselves they love to sleep with the windows open even in winter. Mixed P types do not find heat so intolerable, but usually do prefer cold climates.

K types are *stable* enough not to be greatly disturbed by any extreme of climate, but if pressed often admit they prefer warm weather and are not overfond of high humidity.

SEX DRIVE

V types think a lot about sex. Sometimes they find their fantasies so satisfying that they lose interest in physical consummation. When they are interested, it is intense. Their passion becomes quickly inflamed and peaks quickly as they spend their available energy in the sex act. As with their other appetites their sexual appetite *varies* from day to day, though Vs do tend to fall into habits of sexual overindulgence which leave them exhausted. Their fertility tends to be lower than average.

P people, being *hot-blooded*, usually have ample sexual desire. They know what they want and readily put their desires into action. Whether their desire is great or small, however, Ps are able to balance desire with its fulfillment. If their sexual gratification is thwarted or delayed their innate anger tends to flare up. They are average in fertility.

K individuals experience *steady* desire and normally enjoy sex without being particularly fascinated by it because of their innate reluctance to "spend" energy. Once sex captures their attention, however, their appetite for sex intensifies greatly. They are aroused to passion slowly but remain passionate for a long time once aroused. Their fertility is usually excellent.

PHYSICAL STRENGTH AND ENDURANCE

V types are very active and often restless, but tend to display low stamina. Vigorous exercise tires them quickly—it *dries* them out—and makes them feel hungry afterwards. Unfortunately they often drive themselves to excess and exhaustion through overactivity because they are convinced that "more is better," and because they love to expend energy when they have it. They may become addicted to vigorous exercise because it temporarily makes them feel stable and pain-free. Their muscle tone is usually poor and they must give active attention to developing muscle coordination.

P people can endure vigorous exercise so long as it does not *overheat* them. Ps usually feel both hungry and thirsty after a good workout. They can pace themselves well if they want to, but often do not want to because they are naturally compulsive and competitive. Their muscle tone and coordination are median.

K types have excellent muscle tone and are naturally coordinated. Of all constitutional types they are best able to endure vigorous exercise, but many times are least interested in it because of their aversion to energy expenditure. Once motivated, though, they get great benefit from regular activity, and enjoy it because it makes them feel good. They rarely feel hungry after exercise.

PULSE

Pulse testing should be done early in the morning before eating. You should sit quietly with your back straight and your hands on your thighs for five to ten minutes before you test your pulse, breathing deeply and regularly so that the reading will be accurate. It is usually best to use your radial pulse, the pulse at your wrist below your thumb. Only three of your fingers are necessary for testing: your index, middle and ring fingers. Put your index finger closest to your thumb and your ring finger furthest away from your thumb, toward your elbow.

A V pulse is thin, shallow and *fast* with a broken or *variable* rhythm, or a tendency to skip an occasional beat. In purely V people this pulse seems to slither like a snake, and the artery will feel hard and cool or cold to the touch. It is felt strongest under the index finger.

A P pulse is full, regular, and strong, with medium speed and rhythm; in purely P individuals it often seems to jump like a frog. The artery feels *warm* and soft. It is felt strongest under the middle finger.

The K pulse is strong, full, *slow* and rhythmic like the swimming of a swan, and the artery may feel cool and rubbery. It is felt strongest under the ring finger.

SLEEP

Usually light sleepers, V people may toss and turn and have trouble getting to sleep, or may wake up several times during the night for no apparent reason. Their ability to sleep *varies* greatly from night to night. On some nights, especially when they are exhausted, they will fall into such a deep, prolonged sleep that they are inert to the world and are almost impossible to arouse. Otherwise they are easily disturbed by outside noises because their minds continue to use energy even when they should be resting. Often, no matter how deep or prolonged their sleep, they wake up in the morning feeling unrested for this reason. Frequent sleep-walking and sleep-talking are also indicative of Vs. People who grind their teeth at night are usually V types.

Ps go to sleep easily, sleep lightly and wake up alert. Even when they wake up during the night they can return to slumber quickly. Most nights they enjoy restful sleep, and can get by very well on a minimum of sleep for many nights in a row without seeming ill effect. When they do have trouble sleeping it is usually because of overattention to their work.

K types drop off to sleep quickly and sleep *heavily*, but wake up rested and alert. If permitted, they will gladly sleep many hours at a time, because they save energy that way. Rarely does a K person have difficulty sleeping.

DREAMS

V types dream a lot and forget their dreams easily. In the morning they know they have dreamed but may only be able to remember fragments. Sometimes periods of seeming "dreamlessness" alternate with days or weeks of vivid dreaming. When they do remember, they often report violent, intense, active dreams. *Motion*, particularly flying in the air, is typical of V dreams, as is being pursued by something or someone.

P people can usually remember what they dream. Their dreams are often passionate or otherwise intense, and often involve heat, light, or other energy. Usually the P individual is in control of the dream situation; if there is pursuit, it is usually the P person pursuing and not the other way round. Even dreams of buying and selling are P-type dreams, because they involve transfer of money ("green" energy). P people usually dream in color.

K people usually have very cool, calm, quiet, collected, uneventful, peaceful dreams, like those of an English countryside with cucumber sandwiches at afternoon tea in a gazebo on a swan lake. Ks usually do not bother to remember such dreams; they are more likely to recall those which are intensely emotional.

VOCAL QUALITIES

Untutored V people frequently speak in a breathy voice which becomes hoarse easily and cracks on strain. Voice training may overcome these natural defects. They tend to speak *quickly*, often with rising pitch at the end of a phrase, and tend to stray from the subject. They are usually very talkative and can speak on most any subject to most any audience, even if it is only the cat, the plants or a wall. They speak for the love of speaking. Talking expends a lot of energy, which is one rea-son they love it so. Their conversations may resemble monologues, in fact, two V people can spend hours talking at, not to, one another and both be satisfied afterwards without having communicated much. Part of their vocal weakness results from this overuse of their voices.

P people are usually concise and one-pointed in what they say. They know what they want to communicate, what response they want to eli-cit and how much and what kind of energy needs to be projected to ob-tain the desired response. A P voice frequently carries in it a tone of impatience with the listener, and is usually intense; a P whisper can be clearly heard across a room. Two Ps are sure to communicate with one another, and usually convert a conversation into a contest of wills to see who can outdebate whom. Ps are often accused of having *sharp* tongues.

K types speak *slowly* and cautiously, without volunteering much. In-formation may have to be drawn out of them. A pure K will initiate a conversation only if he or she has something important to say, in con-trast with Vs who will strike up conversations with anyone, and Ps who will approach anyone who seems interesting. K voices tend to be lower in pitch and intensity than the others, but are usually more sonorous and melodious. Ks are a pleasure to listen to when you can get them to talk. Two Ks can easily sit across from one another for hours or days without anything more than a few perfunctory pleasantries passing be-tween them. Perhaps their innate taciturnity helps preserve the sweet-ness of their voices.

CHARACTERISTIC EMOTION

This question concerns how you typically react when you are con-fronted by a stressful situation. You may not actually display this emo-tion if you have taught yourself not to, but your very first reaction is characteristic of your constitution.

For example, once a friend of mine was in a bank when a robber walked in, pointed a gun at him, and said, "Hands up, you goof!"

Vs characteristically show *fear* or anxiety first, which is created by the *dryness* of their inherent Astringency. In such a situation a V type would put his or her hands up immediately.

P types, full of the *heat* of Pungency, ignite into *anger* first, whether they show it outwardly or merely burn with it internally. P types in this situation would raise their hands slowly, thinking only of when they could have their revenge on the gunman.

K people like to avoid confrontations because of the *complacency* of their innate Sweet. They have a strong disinterest in change, and their emotional sensitivity often shows when stressed by unpredictable situa-tions. Like ostriches, they hope that by ignoring a situation it will go away. It takes a lot to arouse them, but once aroused they may feel great fear or anger.

My friend displayed the K response: he first experienced hurt at being called a goof, and then decided to have nothing to do with such an insulting man. He walked out the door of the bank, leaving the astonished bandit gaping behind him. A few yards down the sidewalk, as the emotion wore off, he realized that a robbery was in progress and called the police, who succeeded in nabbing the thief.

PERSONALITY TRAITS

V types are sensitive, high-strung and react quickly to changes in their environments. They are exceptionally *changeable*, and resist regularity in their lives because their active minds demand continual stimulation. When their energy is high they can be the life of the party, but burn out quickly. Sometimes they crave companionship, and other times demand solitude. They usually make friends easily, but their friendships are often short-lived. They love to travel for fun. Their hyperadaptibility gives them flexibility and a potential for detachment, but also tends to make them chaotic and "spacey." They find it difficult to concentrate on any one subject, and often fail to complete the projects they start.

V types recognize the need for self-development but are rarely consistent with any one program. They can become fanatic followers of cults or other far-out doctrines, but even their fanaticism is impermanent, and they may quickly and for little reason switch allegiance to a completely new set of ideas. Their faith often arises from insecurity.

P types are strong and forceful in their dealings. They are dedicated to the practical side of life. When permitted, they are domineering. They are inherently courageous and believe in fair play, and in a good mood exude exuberance, but when angry they can be cruel and hurtful. They make friends easily, especially if their perceive that such friends will be useful to them. They are usually acutely intelligent and tend to be *impatient* with anyone whose intelligence is not equally acute. Their innate arrogance of cleverness can make them intolerant.

P types are dedicated to their own self-development, which sometimes becomes a sort of ego-expansion. Their opinions are strongly held, and they can fall into fanaticism. They tend to stick with their fanatic ideas if they calculate that such a course would benefit them. Cult leaders and their lieutenants are usually P types.

Ks are predominantly calm, quiet, steady, serious sorts who most enjoy the pleasures of home and family. Patience, fortitude and humility are common K virtues. In excess these traits may engender passivity, attachment, possessiveness and greed. K people usually have very *stable* personalities, so stable that they sometime stabilize themselves right out of mental acuity or agility. They study each subject cautiously before committing themselves. Once committed to a course of action, though, they usually see it stubbornly through. They often make friends slowly, after deliberation, but a friendship established usually lasts.

Innate self-satisfaction makes K types less motivated for self-development than others. They do not make good fanatics, but their faith in
whatever they believe is steady and unshakable, though it is often motivated by a desire to maintain the status quo. K types do tend to be innately more compassionate than others, however. Perhaps they are more
maternal because of the strong influence of the Earth Element in their
characters. Mother Earth is Herself mainly Kapha in prakruti.

PREDOMINANT MODE OF EXPRESSION

You can test your predominant sense by remembering your most recent vacation trip; say, for example, to the seacoast. Remember the experience; then ask yourself which aspect of the experience did you first
remember. You may have taught yourself to organize your knowledge
in a specific way, but your first reaction—your prakruti—usually reflects
your constitution.

V types have an acute sense of hearing, so acute that sometimes loud
or dissonant noise can be physically painful to them. They usually first
remember sounds, like the screeching of gulls or the rumble of waves.
V people most often think predominantly in words, and even when they
visualize (thinking in images) or emote (thinking in feelings), they usually use words to tie their thinking together.

P types are visually oriented. They tend to primarily remember images, such as the whitecaps on the breakers or the glare of sunlight on
sand. Ps visualize almost everything they think about and have no difficulty in creating fantasy images. Even if they have been trained to be
very verbal, they always tend to see what they think about, and to use
images to relate words and emotions together.

K people can easily remember the sensations of the sun's heat on
their bodies, or the water's wetness and motion against them as they
swam. Their feelings are emotional as well as physical, and emotions
often influence their thinking as much as or more than the physical "feel"
of things. They often think with their emotions, and "feel" the connection between words and forms.

THE MIND

Vs are good original theorists because they are not afraid to connect
old thoughts in new ways. Their tendency to flit from idea to idea makes
it difficult for them to make their theories function in practice however.

P people are methodical and efficient at planning and the implemen-
tation of the new ideas dreamed up by more theoretical types. Ps love
to engineer ideas into practical uses, and have little interest in the day-
to-day detailed running of a project or business.

K types are stabilizers. They are not renowned either for theorizing
or engineering, but give them a new enterprise and they will run it
smoothly. This sometimes translates into inflexibility or resistance to

change, but if you have a factory or an office to run you will want a K in charge of it.

MEMORY

Vs usually remember easily and forget easily. When angered, they react just like a bottle of soda which is shaken and then opened: they erupt quickly, projecting all their energy into the anger, and as quickly return to normal when their attention is shifted from whatever it was that angered them. Within a short period of time they even forget why they were angry, unless whoever they blew up on reminds them.

Ps usually remember easily and forget with difficulty. When slighted, a P-type will explode with rage, and even after the fire burns itself out the indignation will continue to smoulder for a long, long time. Ps often calculate their energy expenditure so that they can remain angry longer.

Ks need to be told a thing more than once before it sinks in, but once they have learned it they know it for life. Like the elephant, they never forget. Also like the elephant, it takes a good deal to irritate them, but once angered, K types never forget a slight.

LIFESTYLE

Vs find it difficult to create habits of any sort, even those associated with such naturally habitual behavior as eating and sleeping. Financial responsibility is not natural to them. Their innate diffuseness makes it easy for money to get spent as soon as it comes into their hands. They are prone to impulse spending on things they don't really need; money ("green" energy) to them is something meant to be spent.

Ps plan and organize well, calculate their expenditures wisely, and spend sensibly. They are not afraid to spend money but rarely fall prey to impulsive spending. They spend to further specific purposes, and tend to feel superior to those people who cannot exercise such self-control. They make or break habits according to their perception of the habit's utility to them.

Ks enjoy habits, sometimes to the extent of digging themselves into ruts. They always have money saved for that rainy day and can veer toward miserliness. They sometimes indulge in emotional spending, but usually feel that money is meant for accumulation.

Summaries of Constitutional Types

Count the number of V answers, P answers and K answers which you have obtained from this evaluation. Normally, one or two will predominate, and those indicate your prakruti. For example, if you had 9 Vs, 13 Ps, and 3 Ks, your constitution is likely to be P predominant with V secondary. If there is confusion, consider especially your responses to these categories: body frame, skin color and complexion, head hair, appetite, digestion and evacuation, climate preference, dreams, characteristic emotion, and lifestyle.

If you are still confused, think about your preference for temperature. If you really hate cold, and much prefer to be warm, your major predominance is very likely to be Vata. If you truly cannot bear to be too hot, and enjoy the cold for that reason, your are probably predominantly Pitta. And if you are not overtroubled by either, you are likely to have a substantial amount of Kapha in you, even if it is sometimes overshadowed by Pitta or Vata. The summaries below may help you confirm your estimation of your own constitution:

VATA

V types are usually thin and have trouble gaining weight except when they overeat fanatically, which they may do to help stabilize themselves or to provide more energy for the next round of activity. Their bodies are usually narrow in the shoulders and hips and their joints often make a cracking noise when they move them. They tend to be fidgety; fidgeting, like obesity, runs in families.

V people are dry. Their skin usually chaps easily and is prone to corns and calluses. Their hair tends to be coarse, dry and curly. V people suffer from cold, and often complain of poor circulation in their extremities. Their skin is usually cool or cold to the touch. They sweat little and love to be out in the sun.

Their appetites are irregular, and their love for excitement tends to lead them into irregular food habits which worsen their digestion. They usually suffer from or have suffered from chronic constipation, due to innate Astringency. They love soupy, oily, hot foods, but always tend to go to extremes over their food, either indulging in cheesy casseroles and heavy, hard-to-digest items, or denying themselves all heavy foods.

They are prone to rapid fluctuations in their energy levels. Their energy comes in spurts or bursts. Often they try to sustain this energy with Pungent stimulants like coffee rather than admit to themselves that they are tired and need to rest. For a short while they can maintain a level of truly frenzied activity, but exhaustion inevitably follows, which they may not recognize until utter fatigue forces them to rest.

V people often have difficulty with sleep. Either they have trouble falling asleep or staying asleep, or they evade insomnia by maintaining such a high level of exhaustion that whenever they do permit themselves some rest they sleep as if dead. They tend to feel pain more intensely than do other types, and loud noise is also less tolerable to them; their nervous systems seem to have less "insulation" than necessary. A Vs innate drive to avoid pain may manifest as fear. Vs adore oil massage because it helps soothe and quiet the overactive nervous system, which reduces their nervous sensitivity and therefore their pain, physical or mental.

V people live erratic lives because they find great difficulty in creating routine. The Bitter Taste makes them eternally interested in tinkering with themselves and their environment. If *changeability* characterizes most of what you do, you are V predominant.

PITTA

Pure Ps are Pungent, which makes them intense, hot, and irritable. They are usually medium in height, weight, and endurance. Their skin is usually light in color and reddens quickly in the sun, after exercise, or when blushing. They sunburn easily, and usually have plenty of freckles and moles. Their hair tends to be straight, and light in color. Everyone whose hair is naturally red is at least partly P.

P people sweat easily because of all that heat stored inside. The Sour and Salty Tastes ensure that their appetites are always good. They love to eat, because food and drink reduce fire's intensity. If they miss a meal they may "consume" some unwary bystander with their stored anger. They love all foods and usually digest well. They have a tendency to loose stools and are rarely constipated.

Ps powerful fire makes the mind acute as well. P types tend to become quickly impatient around slower or less focused individuals. Ps usually sleep well because they feel it is sensible to do so, but if they become obsessed with work they may spend sleepless nights. They apply the same *intensity* and competitiveness to everything they do, in work or play, and the Pungent Taste makes them anger easily, even if they don't outwardly lose their tempers.

KAPHA

The K type is usually a heavyset individual who is a natural athlete when exercising properly, and who gains weight just by looking at food when neglecting exercise. Most Ks are healthy most of the time, especially if they do not overeat. Ks really do not feel the intense physical hunger that Vs or Ps do, since the Sweet Taste is innately strong in their constitutions, but they can become attached to food as a means of emotional fulfillment. K people sleep soundly and tend to oversleep.

K people generally do not crave the same excitement and stimulation that V and P people love, even from sex, although once they are stimulated the Sour and Salty Tastes become more predominant in them and their appetites awaken. K people are stable, somewhat slow, and tend to be complacent. Attachment to a stable, enjoyable status quo makes K people averse to change and may lead them to become greedy, stubborn, or reactionary. Ks need motivation and stimulation just as Vs require balance and relaxation and Ps require a challenge.

Individuals whose constitutions reflect the influence of only one Dosha are really lucky in the sense that once they know themselves they can always know how they will react to specific stimuli. People with dual constitutions—VP, PK and VK—have personalities which are always in a sense "split": under certain conditions one Dosha will predominate, and under other conditions the other Dosha comes to the fore. The inherent cohesion of personality which characterizes purely V, P or K people is more difficult to come by for those of us who have dual personalities, because we have to try to balance the demands of two very dissimilar principles. Most individuals are dual in constitution.

VATA-PITTA

VP people generally have the poor circulation and love of heat that characterize Vs, but their P nature sets definite limits to their ability to endure heat. The P in them makes them love to eat, but the V ensures they will have trouble digesting large meals. Many of their characteristics show a combination of V and P; for example, they often have wavy hair, caused by a combination of Vs curliness and Ps straightness.

All too often, though, the influences of V and P alternate in the VP individual. When a VP is imbalanced, fear alternates with anger as a response to stress. This can lead to bullying and domineering. The P aspect feels the need to command, but the V aspect creates self-doubt about the individual's capacity or fitness for command, so the compromise involves the domination of beings weaker than oneself.

A healthy, balanced VP weds Vs capacity for original thought and Ps expertise at application of theory. V and P have *lightness* and intensity as their common qualities. Proper direction of this intensity calls for harnessing the lightness for intensive self-development. Otherwise the V tendency toward addiction for pain control and the P predilection for addiction to amplified intensity will drag the VP individual into deeper states of addiction than either V or P people can separately know. VP types most need *stability*. They need to be weighted down with the heaviness which characterizes Kapha, the least influential factor in their personality equation. The Sweet Taste is most important for them.

PITTA-KAPHA

PK people probably adjust best of any constitution to the confusion, irregularity and constant change which characterizes today's world because they combine Ks stability and Ps adaptability. Many of the people who achieve all-round success in life are PKs. Ps active metabolism balances Ks powerful physique to promote good physical health, and Ps anger is well tempered by Ks cautiousness to encourage good mental balance. Though PKs usually prefer temperate climates they can easily endure extremes of heat or cold. They enjoy and profit by vigorous exercise, including sex.

The dark side of the PK individual arises from the shared *oiliness* or wetness of P and K. The ease with which they succeed in the world promotes Ps arrogance and overconfidence and Ks smug self-satisfaction, which can insulate the personality totally and efficiently from all realities other than the reality it wishes to perceive. This is where the oiliness fits in; like "water off a duck's back" criticism may pass unregarded and only flattery may be acknowledged. This attitude can make a successful PK very difficult to live with. Because Vata is minimized in them naturally, PKs need the *dryness* of introspection or spiritual discipline, and the irregularity of exposure to unpredictable situations to prevent overconfidence. Bitter and Astringent are their best Tastes.

VATA-KAPHA

Vata and Kapha are united in their *coldness*. Though they do not suffer as intensely from physical cold as do pure V types because of the strength and insulation of K, they have a double emotional need for heat. They tend to be tall but are average in build and most other physical qualities, just as P types are. Their lack of heat usually manifests physically as digestive disturbances, especially constipation; respiratory disease with much mucus production is also common.

VKs are usually zealous about what they do, and often overdo things by neglecting to use discretion. They can be by turns light, open and airy, and deep and secretive. Their lack of a strong Pitta fire makes personality integration especially difficult for them, because of the diametrically opposite natures of V and K. They must be especially wary of jumping to conclusions without proper preliminary investigation. The deeply emotional nature of K mated with the overactivated up-and-down nature of V ensures that emotional hurt goes deep and remains deep in a VK individual. VKs need *warmth* more than anything else, and they should use the "hot" Tastes (Sour, Salty and Pungent), not exclusively but in preference to the "cold" Tastes (Sweet, Bitter and Astringent).

Constitutions do not change, but perceptions may. After some time you may return to this evaluation and discover that your original opinion about your constitution was inaccurate. This is normal, because as we become healthier our perception of reality becomes less distorted, and what may have seem impenetrably incomprehensible before suddenly becomes profoundly pellucid. Use today's evaluation as the basis for planning your current health strategy. Even if you have erred today in determining your constitution, living for a while according to your current condition will be therapeutic.

The idea of constitutional types is simple, but not simplistic. Every individual has a body and mind which is quite unlike that of any other. Constitutional types do not bind you down into a stereotype; they provide you information on metabolic tendencies which are so deeply ingrained in you that they must be actively balanced if you are to remain in balance. They are simple ways to help you provide a foundation on which you can build the edifice of a new you. Vimalananda always said that if the foundation was good the structure would be good, and if the foundation was imperfect no amount of building could save the structure built on it. Constitution is the start of a road which progresses into more complex, esoteric avenues of personal enhancement.

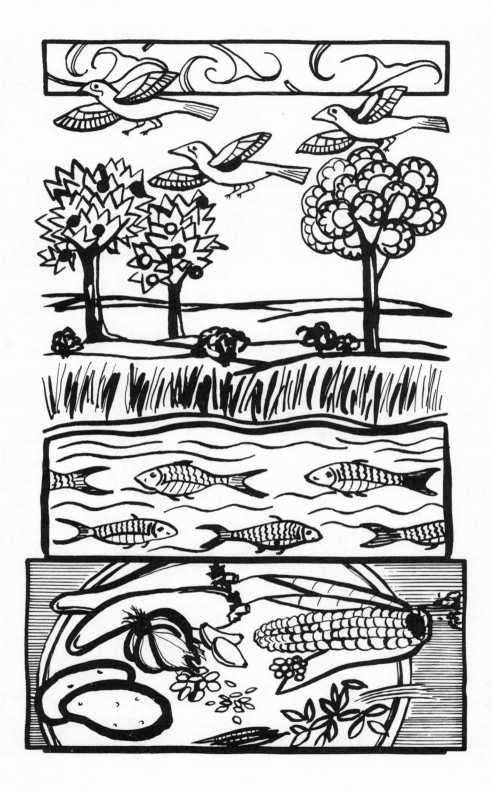

Chapter Three

Food

Ayurveda teaches that food is the Prana, or life force, of living beings, and that life is a continual search for food. "Life lives off life," in the words of a Sanskrit proverb: we maintain our own lives by consuming other living beings.

In Nature's eyes all beings have an equal right to exist. If we wish to remain in harmony with Nature our slaughter of Her children should not be lightly performed. The taking of another's life, even that of a cauliflower, is an act which should be performed with sincere attention to its meaning. Sir Jagadis Chandra Bose, the famous plant physiologist and physicist from India, proved more than fifty years ago that vegetables have sense organs which continue to function even after they leave the vine. According to the ancients, the carrot you crush for juice and the cabbage you chop to cook both feel pain and terror at being slaughtered and dismembered, just as any animal would. Plants cannot communicate their feelings to us, so we wrongly assume they have none. Vegetables and fruits have feelings too.

Few of us live our lives in a way that would make proud the turnip that was tormented for the table, or the radish who relinquished its own identity to become an integral part of you or me. Eating is a sacred act, an offering made into the internal digestive fire for propitiation of the indwelling spirit of a human form in much the same way as offerings are made into external sacrificial fires to propitiate cosmic forces which have been personified into the forms of deities. Since it is a form of worship, eating should be ritualized to emphasize its sacramental aspect.

Each morsel of ingested food must give up its own individual existence and be transmuted so that it can participate in the greater existence of the human body. It is a mystery, and a miracle: that which is "not-you" is converted by Ahamkara into that which is part of you. Undigested food material which escapes into the body cavity causes an inflammatory reaction, but food material which is first digested and assimilated meekly undergoes adaptation into new body parts.

Any substance can act as food, medicine or poison for Ahamkara. Food is that which nourishes the body, mind and spirit. Medicine improves the digestion to enhance nourishment. Poison impedes digestion and disturbs nutrition. Food is anything which you can dominate; medicine is anything which assists you in your domination; poison is anything which challenges this domination.

Some neurotics use food to provide them a sense of accomplishment, a macho sense of having successfully dominated, destroyed and assimilated another being. If in the outside world they are powerless, at the mercy of stronger beings who force them to act against their will, they are still the lords and masters of their private inner worlds and of all food-beings which enter therein. Ritualization of eating helps limit this "bullying" aspect of the personality by automatically abasing the self-congratulating personality in the presence of the Infinite.

Each food article you eat alters your mental disposition. You are naturally attracted to those foods which create within you the state of mind which you desire, and naturally repulsed by those foods which produce opposing states of mind. Some foods, especially those derived from animal flesh, encourage your personality in its bullying and make it want to consume and dominate more and more. Beef and pork are the worst of all foods in this respect. Other foods, including especially milk, grains, raw fruits, and vegetables, help to satisfy this unnatural craving and make you more willing to submit to the will of Nature.

The Ritual of Eating

Begin with your morning routine, paying particular attention to your urine, feces, and tongue. Your urine should be clear and beer-colored, and your feces should be light brown with the consistency of a ripe banana. If your urine is turbid with a foul odor, or your feces is full of undigested food, offensive in odor and passed with abundant gas, Ama is present. Any coating on your tongue also shows that there is Ama, toxins due to improperly digested food, in your digestive tract.

When these signs of Ama, or other signs like nausea or heaviness of the limbs, appear, fast for the day, or at least skip a meal. Do not eat when you are not physically hungry. If you are not sure whether you have ever been physically hungry, a day's fast will teach you what hunger is.

Do not eat when angry, depressed, bored, or otherwise emotionally unstable, or immediately after any physical exertion.

Bathe, or at least wash your hands, face and feet, before you begin.

Sit while eating, in an isolated, clean, area. Face east if possible, the direction of the sun, the Earth's source of heat and fire. Eat alone, or with people you know and trust. Ensure that all your sense organs are satisfied by providing your dining room with pleasant music, fresh flowers, and the like.

Avoid habitual use of restaurants. Most people who sell you food are more concerned with their own profits than with your digestion. Satiation is not determined by how much you eat. A small amount of food presented to you lovingly will satisfy your soul, whereas large heaps of food from a fast-food restaurant may temporarily fill your belly but will leave your mind and spirit unsatisfied.

Only someone who loves you should be permitted to cook for you. Cooks in India are often selected from the priestly class so that there is at least some chance that while cooking some spiritually uplifting vibrations may be transferred into the food. Women should not cook when they are menstruating because they are undergoing a cleansing process and should be relaxing instead.

It is best if your right nostril functions when you eat, since it increases your digestive fire. You can cause it to function by lying on your left side for a few minutes before the meal, by plugging your left nostril, by closing your left nostril with the middle finger of your right hand and breathing rhythmically through your right nostril for a few minutes, or by hooking your left arm over the back of a chair.

Once all is in readiness, pray. Give thanks to Nature for providing you with food, and thank whichever deity you worship for being alive to eat it. Approach each food item with reverence and love, even if you are served something which you dislike but must eat. Suppose your mother-in-law, whom you dislike, serves you rutabagas, which you hate. If wishing to maintain family peace you eat the rutabagas under duress, those vegetables will carry your dislike and hatred deep into your system and disturb your balance. Consume your food, even if you dislike it, with respect for the sacrifice it is making for you, and it will carry the harmonizing power of your prayer inside you instead.

Before you begin your meal, feed someone else. Traditionally in India a five-fold offering is made: to the sacred fire, a cow, a crow, a dog, and another human being, who might be a child, a beggar, or anyone else outside one's own family. This is a practical thanks to Nature, a feeding of some of Her children in gratitude to Her for providing you some of Her other children as sacrifices for consumption. And, it is another way of controlling Ahamkara, an admission that the food is intended not for mere self-gratification but for the greater good of all beings. Feed anyone—a pet, a plant, a neighbor, a stranger—so you can experience a little of Nature's joy, the joy which a mother feels when she feeds her children and watches them grow and develop in consequence.

Immediately before beginning to eat, chew some ginger to awaken your taste buds, start your juices flowing, and purify your tongue and mouth. P people should omit this step. It is best to prepare the ginger by slicing it into long thin strips and marinating it in lemon juice with an optional pinch of rock salt.

Concentrate on your meal. No TV, radio, stereo, or conversation should distract your attention. Observe silence while you eat; sit and chat afterwards.

Chew each morsel slowly and attentively many times. When feasible, eat with your hands so that your skin can send temperature and texture cues to your brain.

Feed all five senses by eating food which is attractive to the eye, tasty, aromatic, and pleasing in texture and sound (like the bubbling of a hot casserole or the hiss of a frying pancake).

After eating, drink a mixture of yogurt churned with water to assist digestion. People with weak digestion should use non-fat yogurt and a 1:3 proportion of yogurt to water; those with stronger digestion may use normal yogurt in a proportion of up to 3:1 yogurt to water. V people should add lemon juice and a pinch of salt, and spice the mixture with fresh diced ginger or chilies, or whole or powdered cumin and coriander; P people should use coriander leaf or seed or cardamom powder, with less lemon juice and some sweetener like maple syrup or even sugar; K people should use honey with powdered ginger or black pepper, or other hot spices like diced green chilies. Anyone who is allergic to dairy products should omit this step, and some authorities suggest that all dairy products should be avoided at a meal in which flesh is consumed.

At the end of the meal again give thanks, clean your mouth, apply water to your eyes to prevent weakening of vision because of increased Pitta at this time, urinate but do not encourage defecation, and then take a brief walk of 100 steps to promote digestion.

Avoid exercise or sex within an hour of food, and sleeping or studying within two hours. If you have overeaten, or if you are physically weak, lie for a few minutes without going to sleep on your left side to insure that your right nostril is working well to keep your digestion hot.

Avoid eating too late at night. Do not eat any Kapha-producing food like melons, yogurt, sesame products, cheese or ice cream at night. Generally, all ice-cold food weakens digestion.

Ks should eat only twice a day, allowing at least a six-hour gap between meals and should not snack. Ps should eat three meals daily with gaps of four to six hours between them. They may snack if they retain a consistent four-hour gap. Vs should always eat small meals three or four times a day and may snack as needed with gaps of at least two hours. No one should allow less than two hours between any two meals or snacks because the gut requires at least this much time to ready itself for the next food.

The Qualities of Food

All food is either light or heavy for digestion. Light foods include rice, mung beans, and wild meats like venison. Heavy foods include milk, black beans, raw fruits and vegetables, beef and pork. Cooking and preparation can alter these qualities; for example, milk becomes lighter when heated with saffron, and rice is made heavier by cooking with milk.

In general animal flesh is heavier than vegetables, legumes or grains; raw food is heavier than cooked, and preserved food is heavier than fresh. Raw food and cooked food should not be consumed together at the same meal, excepting small amounts of raw foods as appetizers or chutneys with a cooked meal, or small amounts of sauces or dressings on a raw meal. Do not mix heavy and light foods at the same meal; do not mix fresh food with leftovers. Very hot and very cold substances, like Mexican food and ice cream, should not be consumed together at the same meal.

Light food assists the mind's efforts to integrate body, mind and spirit because it pulls less blood down into the body during the digestive process. Heavy food requires more energy input to be digested, so more blood is drawn into the gut and less remains for the brain to use. Rice is light, wheat is heavy. The wheat-eaters of North India are proud that they are more massively built than the rice-eaters of Southern India. The Southern Indians counter with accurate smugness that "wheat increases brawn, but rice increases brain." According to the Bhagavad Gita, the food articles which most increase mental equilibrium when they are eaten in appropriate quantities and properly digested are rice, mung beans, milk, ghee, honey, and pure water.

You may eat to your fill, but not beyond, of light food, but you must not eat more than one-half the quantity of any heavy food you might desire. People who are weak or ailing or sedentary or do not exercise should not take more than one-half their capacity of any solid food, no matter how light it is, and should take one-fourth their capacity as liquid. The remaining one-fourth of the stomach should be left empty to allow room for proper mixing of digestive juices with nutrients. Some authorities suggest that these proportions should be equal thirds.

V people are more likely to require cooked food than P people, who often do best on raw food. It is rare to find pure Vs who can balance themselves on a purely raw food diet, whereas P or PK people can live almost indefinitely on raw food. VP people can usually exist comfortably on raw food during the spring and summer. Raw food helps tone up the digestive tract for K and VK people, but lack of intrinsic fire means that such people can overdo raw food.

V people do best of all on one-pot meals: soups, stews, casseroles, and the like. In a stew, all the ingredients—meat, grain, legume, vegetable—lose their own individuality and are welded into a single substance. Taken separately, each separate food demands different digestive attention from the body. Such foods may fight over this attention once they are inside the gut, causing indigestion.

This is why food combining is more important for V people than it is for other types. The V digestive system is not capable of handling a variety of foods at once, no matter how small the quantity, because the dryness and variability of Vata limits digestive responsiveness. Irregularity in diet disturbs Vata, and worsens digestion further. In a one-dish meal, however, the various foods have settled their differences in the pot, fought out whatever needed to be fought out, and come to some conclusion, which you then consume. One-pot meals are best for everyone during illness, convalescence, and rejuvenation therapy.

Avoid all food articles which have been wrongly prepared, such as those which have honey baked into them, or which are overcooked, undercooked, burnt, unpleasant tasting, unripe, overripe, putrefied, stale, and otherwise revolting. Fried food aggravates all three Doshas. Vata increases because of the dryness developed during the frying process, Pitta increases because of the heat of the frying process and the rancid oiliness of the resulting food, and Kapha increases because of the heaviness of the oil and the stickiness of the food after frying. Fried food also impairs the eyesight, and should not be eaten regularly.

Every food you eat affects your mind as well as your body. The mind has three possible states:

Sattva, or *equilibrium*, the mind's normal state in which it discriminates accurately;

Rajas, or *motion*, a state in which excessive mental activity weakens discrimination; and

Tamas, or *inertia*, a state in which insufficient mental activity weakens discrimination.

Food which is putrid or vile in taste, or which is fermented, like alcohol, or has been preserved for too long, promotes Tamas. Legumes and other high-protein food like meat, fish, and fowl increase Rajas, as do Pungent spices. Rajas and Tamas disturb mind-body-spirit integration. Sattva, which promotes this integration, is promoted by Sweet foods like grains and fruits, and some vegetables and dairy products.

Garlic and onions are both Rajasic and Tamasic, and are forbidden to Yogis because they root the consciousness more firmly in the body. However, if you are already imbalanced it is wise to use garlic, onions, and other such substances to improve your body-consciousness before you try to follow strict spiritual food discipline.

Eat food directly from the farm as often as possible. Besides offering superior freshness and taste, such produce has been through fewer hands to get to you. The food we buy in our cities has passed through the hands of the farmer, the dealer, the wholesaler, and the retailer before reaching our tables. Each of these worthies has dealt with the food from a profit-making motive, not as a sacrament for sacrifice, and have thereby added negativity to the food. All negativity in your food disturbs your mind.

Eating habits affect digestive capability. For example, if you always eat cooked food, the day you eat raw food you will find it hard to digest because your system is not used to it. Some habits are good: the regular use of rice, wheat, barley, mung beans, daikon radish, ginger, onions, garlic, grapes, pomegranates, buttermilk or churned yogurt, ghee, rock salt and pure water is good for anyone whose constitution permits them. P people, for instance, should not make the use of garlic habitual, since it is too hot for them. Wild game is the only meat which is good for regular use.

Food articles to which you should *never* become habituated because they are too heavy to be properly digested include unchurned yogurt, pork, beef, mutton, dried meat, dried vegetables, molasses, and cheese, as well as any foods which are very cold, very hot, thoroughly tasteless, or too intense in taste.

Although meat is mandated in Ayurveda for debilitated patients, for warriors and for those who overexert themselves, it is very heavy for digestion, putrefies faster than other foods and produces Ama quickly. Unless you exercise strenuously, regular meat eating will increase Fat rather than Flesh. It promotes speed rather than endurance, which is not good for Vata-affected individuals. Meat overheats the mind and warms the body, but even in cold climates it should not be used to excess. Today's meat is also of poor quality, full of antibiotics and other drugs, taken from feedlot animals who never exercise so that all their Ama remains in their tissues.

Esoterically, the fear felt by the animal as it waits to be slaughtered and the hatred it feels for the human who slaughters it change the composition of its flesh and increase fear and anger in whoever eats it. The more the violence involved in the collection of our food, the greater the violence in our lives. Also, because digestive wastes are partly excreted in sweat, a meat-eater sits in his or her own body odor daily, breathing in chemicals which promote fear and anger, and projecting this fear and anger out at others.

Foods for Each Constitution

Every food substance has its own personality, a Taste personality, which interacts with your consciousness and affects it. These effects, like those of meat, are complex and not easily knowable in full. The knowledge of a food's Taste, Energy and Post-Digestive Effect makes it easier to predict these effects, although there are also other qualities which influence the result. The observations made below are conditional on your individual condition: your food allergies, digestive capacity, and present degree of Dosha aggravation. The nectar of immortality itself is poison to anyone who cannot digest it. The food items listed below after each constitutional type are those items which are usually good for that constitution. The lists are not exclusive.

FOODS FOR VATA CONSTITUTIONS

Sweet, Sour and Salty foods are generally good for V people, since they satisfy the system and reduce its insecurity about being well fed. Bitter, Pungent and Astringent foods are less beneficial because they dry the system and intensify emotional instability, especially insecurity. Large amounts of any Taste should be avoided because Vata is aggravated by excess.

Grains - Of all grains wheat is most satisfying to Vs, but it is heavy and easy to become allergic to. Well-cooked oats and rice are good. Buckwheat, corn, millet and rye all tend to be drying and therefore not as good for V as the others, but because grain as a category is nourishing and therefore desirable for V people these grains are included as well for variety. They especially must be cooked with plenty of water, and with butter, ghee or oil added to reduce their dryness. Rice gruel is optimal for any whose digestion is catastrophic. Yeasted bread is not a good staple food for V people because fermentation fills it full of gas bubbles. Unyeasted bread is better, but since bread of any sort is somewhat dried out by baking, freshly cooked grains are always better for V types.

Vegetables - Cooked rather than raw vegetables are best for Vata. Even some of the vegetables missing from the V list, like mushrooms, eggplant, peas and spinach, are suitable for V people if they are well-cooked and consumed only occasionally. Others, like onions and okra which are found on the list, often cause difficulties to the V person who consumes them raw. Most rough, hard vegetables like celery are better digested as juices. Salads of leafy greens like parsley, cilantro (coriander leaf, also known as Chinese parsley), lettuce, spinach and sprouts are all good for Vs on occasion if they are eaten with a good oily or creamy dressing.

Cucumbers, the squashes and zucchini can be consumed from time to time if they are cooked well with oil. Tomatoes are not good for Vs when raw, but tomato sauce cooked into a pasta meal, for example, may be suitable because the indigestible tomato skin and seeds have been removed. If a V individual has stiff, aching joints or muscles, which indicate deep-seated Ama, they should definitely avoid spinach, potatoes, tomatoes, eggplant and peppers.

The vegetables which are best for V types include:

Asparagus, Beets, Carrots, Celery, Garlic, Green Beans, Okra, Onion, Parsnips, Radishes, Rutabagas, Turnips, Sweet Potatoes, Water Chestnuts

Fruits - Most fruits are good for Vs, except those which are naturally Astringent like cranberries and pomegranates, or those which are drying, like apples. However, cranberry sauce and pomegranate syrup are acceptable, as are stewed or baked apples or applesauce. Sweet pomegranate juice is permissible. All dried fruits, even the Sweet ones like figs and grapes, are inappropriate for Vs unless they are reconstituted to normal juiciness by soaking in water, or better yet by stewing, which heats them up as well.

Unripe fruits should be avoided, especially bananas, which are Astringent when unripe. Ripe bananas are good, however, because judiciously used they can control either diarrhea or constipation and are soothing to the gut. Mangoes and apricots are especially good. Overuse of melons may cause disturbance of both Vata and Kapha, and can be prevented by eating fennel, clove, black pepper or red pepper on the melon as an antidote.

The fruits which are good for Vs include:

Apricots, Avocados, Bananas, Berries, Cherries, Coconut, Dates, Figs, Grapefruit, Grapes, Lemons, Mangoes, Melons, Nectarines, Oranges, Papaya, Peaches, Pears, Persimmons, Pineapples, Plums

Flesh Foods - Vs are the only people who truly need animal foods in their diet, because they need the complete proteins these animal foods provide. Overindulgence in animal flesh, though, quickly weakens the sensitive V digestion. Even if it is well digested, long-term use of any high-protein food always increases Vata because the residue of protein digestion adds to the body's nitrogenous waste burden.

Many Vs are able to fill their need for animal protein by judicious use of dairy products. Otherwise eggs, chicken, turkey, fresh fish and venison are all generally good for Vs. The only commercially available red meat they should eat is goat or lamb, which sometimes can help provide temporary balance to the system. While goat is good for V people, lamb should not be consumed regularly. Beef is permissible when absolutely necessary to "ground" the V person immediately. Care should be taken with shellfish because of its potential to cause allergies. Eggs should be scrambled, with milk if possible, or poached; fried eggs ought not to be regularly consumed.

Legumes - Legumes are the vegetable kingdom's equivalent of meat. They are high in difficult-to-digest protein, whose metabolic by-product is nitrogenous waste. Nitrogen is a gas, and all gases increase Vata. Nitrogen has even been shown to be essential to the development of certain cancers which hate oxygen. To prevent this, overindulgence in protein should be avoided. Mung beans are the best of all high-protein foods because they are the lightest for digestion and disturb the mind least. Peanuts encourage the blood to clot and should not be eaten by anyone whose circulation is already impared.

Cook legumes with turmeric, to prevent them from toxifying the blood; cumin and coriander seeds, to enkindle the digestive fire; and ginger, garlic or asafoetida to prevent Vata from being disturbed. Add a little oil to the cooking pot for this same Vata-controlling purpose. Increased Vata due to beans and peas usually comes in the form of intestinal gas, and can be reduced by soaking the legume for at least an hour before cooking, and throwing away that water. If they are still too gas-producing, boil the legumes five to ten minutes in an excess of water and discard that liquid before starting to cook them.

In India peas and lentils are most often used split. Splitting exposes more surface of the legume to the cooking process, and eliminates the indigestible outer coat. The best way to use these split pulses is to cook them into a well-spiced soup and consume them with grains. If you cannot locate split peas and beans you can sprout them first and then wash off the hulls.

Vs should eat only a small amount of legume at any one meal. Even tofu, which is pre-digested, can aggravate Vata if consumed daily in large amounts over a long period of time. The best legumes for V people are black lentils, red lentils, chickpeas, mung beans, and tofu. Black lentils are very strengthening but are also very heavy to digest. They must be well soaked before cooking and must be cooked with extra garlic or asafoetida.

Nuts and **Seeds** - Almonds are the best of all nuts. They should never be eaten with their skins, which irritate the lining of the gut, nor should they be blanched in hot water. Soak them overnight and peel them the next morning. Ten almonds each morning provides the body with enough nutrients for the whole day. Pumpkin seeds are a brain tonic. Being heavy for digestion, overuse of sesame products gradually ruins the tone of the gastro-intestinal tract. All nuts and seeds are good for V people, but are too concentrated for regular use unless they are made into nut and seed butters or milks. Overconcentrated food, which resists penetration by digestive juices, is one of the chief causes of Vata-caused indigestion.

Oils - In general, sesame is the best oil, and safflower oil the worst, but all oils are good for V. Almond oil is good for the brain, coconut and sesame oils for the hair, and mustard oil for the skin.

Dairy - All dairy products are good for V types who are not allergic to them. Hard cheeses should be eaten sparingly; because they are so compact and concentrated they should be cooked into a more liquid form, like fondue or chile con queso. Yogurt, blended with water and spiced with ginger, cumin or the like helps remove Vata from the system.

Sweeteners - Sweet reduces Vata. Vs can use any sweetener in moderation except white sugar, which is poisonous for them. Honey may be used freely but must never be cooked. Overuse of Sweet eventually increases Vata.

Spices - All spices, and especially ginger and garlic, are good for Vs and VKs in small quantities. Vs are always tempted to overuse spices, hoping to improve their digestive capacities, but overuse of hot spices eventually aggravates Vata. VP people should be cautious of spices because the V aspect of their natures craves them and the P aspect can be seriously aggravated by them. Asafoetida is one of the best spices for Vata control, but should not be used by anyone with too much heat in the liver or the mind. Cold fennel or sandalwood tea can overcome any ill effect of asafoetida in a V person; pomegranate and apple can be used for other types.

Vices - This category is included because human beings do fall prey to vice now and again. If you are going to sin, you should at least do so wisely, and avoid falling prey to guilt or side-effects. No intoxicating substance should ever be used habitually by anyone.

V people are prone to addiction. They should avoid all vices, including especially tobacco, sugar and caffeine. Half a glass of wine diluted with water, with or after a meal, is beneficial for a V person; larger quantities of alcohol can be deadly. Vs should avoid all wines which are known to have chemical additives. Beer is not so good as wine for Vs because of its yeast content, and hard liquor is too intense for the V constitution. Intensity is itself intoxicating to V people, but intensity encourages erraticalness. Relaxation and meditation are better.

FOODS FOR PITTA CONSTITUTIONS

P people should avoid Sour, Salty and Pungent, the "hot" Tastes, and should concentrate on Sweet, Bitter and Astringent, the "cold" Tastes. If Vs should especially avoid caffeine and sugar, Ps should especially avoid meat, eggs, alcohol and salt. All these substances augment Pitta's natural aggressiveness and compulsiveness. Grains, fruit and vegetables cool the Pitta heat and should form the majority of the P diet. Vegetarianism is best for P people; every P should make a sincere effort to become vegetarian.

Grains - Barley is the supreme grain for P people because it is both cooling and drying, and helps reduce excess stomach acid. Rice comes next, followed by oats and wheat. Buckwheat, corn, millet and rye are all heating and should not be consumed habitually by Ps. Yeasted bread is not good for Pitta because of the Sourness produced during fermentation, but unyeasted breads are good.

Vegetables - Ps can eat vegetables all day long, and should concern themselves only to avoid Sour vegetables like tomatoes and Pungent vegetables like radishes. Tomatoes in all forms are forbidden. Garlic should be avoided. Beets, carrots and the long white radishes called daikon purify the liver and help Ps control Pitta as long as Pitta is not already increased. If Pitta is disturbed they should be avoided.

Steamed white or yellow onions are good on occasion for P people because these onions, even though they are Hot, lose their Pungency on cooking and become wholly Sweet. Red or purple onions are too Pungent for Ps, as are all varieties of peppers. Creamed spinach or spinach with cottage cheese is usually satisfactory for P types. Even normally permitted vegetables like parsley should be avoided if for reasons of age or growing conditions they taste unusually Sour or Pungent. Likewise, even vegetables which are not listed below are permissible when a particular specimen is unusually Sweet.

Ps do best with these vegetables:

Asparagus, Broccoli, Brussels Sprouts, Cabbage, Cilantro, Cucumber, Cauliflower, Celery, Cress, Green Beans, Leafy Greens, Lettuce, Mushrooms, Okra, Peas, Parsley, Potatoes, Sprouts, Squashes, Water Chestnuts, Zucchini

Fruits - Ps should eat Sweet fruits and avoid Sour fruits. Any piece of fruit on the list below which might happen to be Sour should not be eaten; this especially includes apples, cherries, grapes, oranges, pineapples, and pomegranates. Likewise, any fruit like berries which are not on this list may be eaten if they are exceptionally Sweet. Papaya is generally too "hot" for the P constitution. Bananas, even though they are Sweet and reportedly help cure ulcers, have a Sour Post-Digestive Effect and should not be eaten regularly by P types. Figs and grapes are especially good for Ps, since they both are Sweet and act as laxatives. Grapes are the Queen of Fruit, and mangoes are the King. Even though lemons and limes are Sour, they reduce Pitta if used sparingly; overuse, especially of lemons, will however increase Pitta.

The following fruits are best for Ps:

Apples, Apricots, Avocados, Cherries, Coconut, Dried Fruits, Figs, Grapes, Lemons, Mangoes, Melons, Nectarines, Oranges, Peaches, Pears, Persimmons, Pineapples, Plums, Pomegranates

Flesh Foods - P people should not eat seafood at all because it is "hot" and tends to cause allergies. Egg yolks are hot, and egg whites cooling. Ps can digest flesh foods, but should generally avoid them because they pollute the blood and because they encourage aggression and irritability. Chicken, turkey, rabbit, and venison are permissible for P people.

Legumes - P people have less difficulty digesting all foods, but should be wary of legume overconsumption because the same nitrogenous wastes which aggravate Vata also aggravate Pitta because of their acidity. However, in small amounts all legumes except red and yellow lentils are good for them. The best legumes for Ps are black lentils, chickpeas, mung beans, and tofu.

Nuts and **Seeds** - Most nuts and seeds are too hot and oily for P types. Coconut is good for P people because even though it is oily it is also very cooling. Freshly squeezed coconut milk is excellent for aggravated Pitta. Sunflower seeds and pumpkin seeds are also permissible.

Oils - Ps should avoid oils, but may consume small amounts of almond, or larger amounts of coconut, olive or sunflower oils.

Dairy - All Sweet dairy products, like milk, unsalted butter, and ghee, are good for P types; no Sour products are. Yogurt can be consumed if it is spiced with cinnamon or with coriander and a few drops of lemon juice, a sweetener is added, and it is blended with equal parts of water. P people should use soft, unsalted cheeses; hard cheeses should be strictly limited.

Sweeteners - Pitta is relieved by sweets. Of all people Ps can best handle Sweet food, including sugar, because sweets reduce heat. This is why residents of hot countries can eat more sugar and suffer less for it than can residents of colder climes. Molasses is "hot" and Ps should not use it. Long-term overuse of honey, which is also "hot," could theoretically aggravate Pitta.

Spices - Spices increase the typical P aggressive impatience. Ps should resist the temptation to become addicted to hot spices and should use only the cooling spices listed here. Mustard should be eliminated, and salt eliminated or drastically reduced, from the P diet. Cumin, being hot, is always used with coriander for balance. The best spices for regular use by P people are cardamom, cinnamon, coriander, fennel, and turmeric, and small amounts of cumin and black pepper.

Vices - Tobacco is too hot for the P system, as is alcohol. An occasional beer may, however, help a P relax. Black tea is Astringent and may be used occasionally. Coffee is Pungent and irritating to the liver and so must not be used habitually. Prolonged use of coffee weakens the digestive fire, overheats the blood, and produces such symptoms as emaciation, headache, palpitations and breathing difficulty. Treatment for coffee addiction must address both Vata and Pitta, and should employ milk, ghee, and butter freely to antidote its effects.

FOODS FOR KAPHA CONSTITUTIONS

K people need to concentrate on Bitter, Pungent and Astringent food, which invigorate their bodies and minds, and should avoid Sweet, Sour and Salty substances, which help them remain set in their ways. Ks should never eat fried or otherwise greasy food, and should shun dairy products. Fat is the worst possible food for K types. Vegetables are best for Ks, who should limit the total amount of food they eat.

Grains - K people need grain less than do V or P people. The hot, drying grains buckwheat and millet are best for Ks, followed by barley, rice, and corn. K people do best with roasted or otherwise dry-cooked grains. All breads should be toasted, or better yet avoided. Wheat is too heavy, cold and oily to be good for Ks.

Vegetables - All vegetables are good for K except potatoes, tomatoes, and water chestnuts. Cucumbers, though Sweet, are also Bitter and Astringent and therefore do not aggravate Kapha. K people should avoid very Sweet, very Sour, and very juicy vegetables. Otherwise they can eat as many vegetables as they like as often as they like. Leafy greens and vegetables which contain seeds (like squashes) should get preference over root vegetables, which are naturally more Earthy. Raw vegetables are good; steamed or stir-fried vegetables are easier to digest. Peppers are good for K types. K people who overdose on chilies, cayenne, or other hot Pungent spices may use ghee to antidote any resulting Pitta aggravation.

Fruits - K people should avoid both very Sweet and very Sour fruits, and any fruits which are very juicy. Dried fruits like prunes are good. The best fruits for Ks are apples, apricots, cranberries, mangoes, peaches, pears, and pomegranates.

Flesh Foods - K people rarely need any flesh foods because their flesh is adequately nourished by other foods. When they do eat flesh it should be roasted, broiled, baked, or otherwise cooked dry, but never fried. They may eat chicken, eggs, rabbit, seafood, and venison.

Legumes - K people should not overeat legumes any more than they should overeat meat, because their bodies do not require large quantities of protein. Legumes are much better for Ks than meat, though, because of the lack of animal fat. K people should however avoid the heaviest of the legumes, such as black lentils, kidney beans, and soy beans. Well-cooked tofu is permissible for Ks in small quantities; larger quantities are likely to increase Kapha. The best legumes for K people are black beans, mung beans, pinto beans, and red lentils.

Nuts and **Seeds** - K people do not need the heavy, oily energy of nuts and seeds and should avoid them. They may eat sunflower seeds and pumpkin seeds on occasion.

Oils - K people should avoid the use of oils. They may use almond, corn, safflower, or sunflower oils when necessary.

Dairy - K types do not need the heavy, oily, sticky, cooling qualities of dairy products, which are very like Kapha's own qualities. Small amounts of ghee are good, and goat's milk is better than cow's milk because it is "hotter." Goat's milk is good for respiratory diseases in any constitution.

Sweeteners - Kapha is increased by sweets, and Ks should not use any sweeteners except raw honey, which helps reduce Kapha.

Spices - Ks find spices useful to awaken their organisms; they can use all spices except salt, which increases Kapha directly. As for V people, ginger and garlic are best for Ks.

Vices - Only pure K people can really benefit from occasional use of stimulants. Black tea is good for them, and coffee is acceptable. Occasional smoking is not as bad for Ks as it is for Vs or Ps because the heat and subtlety of the smoke can help reduce Kapha. Overindulgence in smoking is certain to increase Kapha, however. K people really do not need to use alcohol at all, but if they do they should avoid beer and drink only wine, or diluted hard liquor. Only pure Ks should ever touch hard liquor.

The above suggestions are guidelines only. You will have to discover for yourself which rules are most important for you to follow and which can be ignored safely on occasion. As far as possible you should avoid the foods which are inappropriate for your prakruti, but when you want to cheat you should cheat at the right time.

P people who want to eat hot spicy food should not do so at noon or in the summer, when Pitta is at its height, but only in the early morning or the early evening, or in the fall or winter when Kapha can cover for them. K types who want to enjoy heavy, sticky food should avoid morning and evening, and winter and spring, and eat it only at noon in the summer when Pitta can help them digest it. Vs should not eat Vata-promoting junk food in the afternoons or in autumn when Vata naturally predominates; they should stick to morning or noon, in spring or summer, when the influence of Kapha or Pitta is greater.

DUAL PRAKRUTIS

Generally a VP person should follow a Vata-controlling diet in fall and winter, and a Pitta-controlling diet in spring and summer. Since Pungent increases both Vata and Pitta and Sweet controls both these Doshas, VPs should especially avoid spicy, Pungent food and the anger they create, and search for Sweetness in everything they do, especially eating.

PK people should follow a Pitta-controlling diet from late spring through early fall, and a Kapha-controlling diet from late fall through early spring. Bitter and Astringent are best for PKs, as are their associated willingness to accept change and lack of security, because both Tastes control both Pitta and Kapha. Sour and Salty, and their envy and hedonism, are doubly dangerous for PK people because both increase both Pitta and Kapha.

VKs should concentrate on controlling Vata in summer and fall and controlling Kapha in winter and spring. Since both Vata and Kapha are cold and need heat, VKs should prefer Sour, Salty and Pungent, the "hot" Tastes, to Sweet, Bitter and Astringent, the "cold" Tastes. In summer and fall Sour and Salty may be preferred but should be balanced with Sweet. In winter and spring Pungent may be preferred but should be balanced with Bitter and Astringent.

Specific Food Items

While brown rice is full of nutrients, polished rice has been used in its place in India since time immemorial. Brown rice is too rough in texture for V people, too hot for P people, and too heavy for K people to use regularly. Basmati rice is good for regular use because it is parboiled before it is polished. This parboiling drives the vitamins and minerals deep into the grain so that only small amounts are lost during the milling process. If you choose to use polished basmati rice either ensure that locally grown varieties were parboiled before polishing, or purchase an imported variety from an Indian grocery store.

Milk is meant for people who have powerful digestion, who are very sexually active, or who are emaciated from some other Vata-producing activity and need rest and sleep. Mung bean soup can be used as a substitute if milk is unavailable or inadvisable. Some Yogis live on milk alone because it is the only food given willingly through joy by any being for the purpose of nourishing another. Its mental side-effects are almost nil, and it encourages motherliness in the drinker. Fruit and honey are also foods which are meant for other beings, but they are not relinquished willingly, and their use by humans may deny their original recipients a chance at life. All other foods, including nuts, seeds and grains, involve the killing of another being.

Milk also helps integrate the consciousness. Other animal protein is derived from flesh and drags the consciousness down into the flesh. It discourages that breaking free of earthly restraints which is required for spiritual advancement. Because it is so different in composition from animal protein, plant protein though healthy is sometimes insufficient to ground the consciousness firmly enough in the physical body. Milk is the one food which combines the Sattvic essence of plants with the firm groundedness of animals.

Some authors argue that milk is useful only for young animals and should not be consumed by adults. While it is true that some people are genetically incapable of digesting milk properly, it is unwarranted to suggest that milk is bad for everyone. The diet of the Masai tribe of Kenya, for example, is almost entirely composed of milk. Although Masais are dreaded as warriors, they never kill the animals of the jungle, and only rarely will they slaughter their cattle for food, because they believe so strongly that all beings have a right to live. Is it possible that centuries of milk consumption have encouraged them in this attitude?

Milk is wrongly blamed for many ills. It should not be:

Drunk cold. Milk is Cold in Energy, and serving it at refrigerator temperatures compounds its coldness and heaviness.

Homogenized. Homogenization changes the fat and makes it almost indigestible, which encourages Ama formation.

Consumed with other food. Milk is a complex, complete food and should be taken alone, or with ghee and honey. It may however be cooked with certain other foods like grains.

Overconsumed. A pint of milk at a sitting is usually more than sufficient for the system to deal with at a time.

Unspiced. A pinch of saffron added to warm milk greatly improves its digestibility. Turmeric and ginger may be used instead, as may cardamom, cinnamon, nutmeg or clove. Even on its own honey reduces milk's tendency to produce Kapha.

Butter is tonic to the brain, especially after it has been clarified into ghee. One tablespoon of melted ghee with half a teaspoon of sugar or maple syrup helps promote mental coolness in P types. Replacing the sugar with a teaspoon of honey helps promote mental cohesion in V types. Ghee increases the digestive fire without increasing Pitta, helps remove the effects of poisons, promotes beauty, improves the complexion and luster, and is aphrodisiac. It promotes mental stability and intelligence, and is a good vehicle for most herbs.

Ghee and honey potentiate each other when taken together, but they should never be mixed in equal quantities. Take more ghee than honey (at least 2:1) if you want improved tissue nutrition, and more honey than ghee (at least 2:1) if increased digestive capacity is your goal.

Honey is both medicine and food. It is a superior medicine because like poison it spreads immediately throughout the whole body and penetrates to the deepest tissues without being first digested. Poison ruins the tissues, but honey, having been predigested to act as food for poisonous baby bees, nourishes them. Honey is good for the heart and the eyes, helps heal wounds when applied to them directly, removes poisons from the body, and transports any herb added to it deep into the tissues. It is also aphrodisiac. Honey should *never* be used in cooking or baking, as extreme heat increases its poisonous qualities and makes it produce Ama in the body. It is better to use barley malt, rice bran syrup, or date sugar for baking.

Salt is intense, hot, heavy and oily. Used in excess it ages the body quickly, increasing wrinkles, baldness and patchy falling of hair, producing diseases of blood and flesh, loosening the muscles and joints, and promoting weakness, lethargy, debilitation, and a decreased capacity to work. Reducing salt in your diet can make you live longer and healthier. P and K people especially should try to eliminate salt from their diets, and Vs should eat just enough salt to keep their digestive fires hot. The best of all salts is Saindhava, a variety of rock salt from the Sindh region of Pakistan which does not cause the body to retain water as most salts do.

Yogurt increases Kapha because its qualities are almost exactly the

same as those of Kapha. Honey reduces yogurt's Kapha-forming qualities, and spices antidote it even further. The addition of water to this
spiced yogurt dilutes it, and churning breaks up its gel structure to make
it less slimy and viscid. The resultant mixture aggravates Kapha very
little and promotes digestion greatly. Everyone who is not allergic to
dairy products should drink a cup of it at the end of each meal.

Addiction and Taste

Humans frequently become habituated to foods which do not agree
with them because of the intoxicating effects such foods have. V people,
for example, often become hypoglycemic because they love to eat sugar,
since sugar provides instant satisfaction and temporarily controls the
mental erraticalness which Vata creates. P people may become habituated to meat or to hot spices which inflame Pitta and make them more
obsessive, intense, goal-oriented and driven. K people may find themselves habituated to heavy, fatty foods which reinforce their natural complacency.

All of us use our food to affect our consciousness; most of us, though,
prefer to perpetuate all our old idiosyncrasies and personality traits, instead of improving them with a diet balanced according to individual
constitution. We live in a fast world in which many of us try to run even
faster than the world forces us to. Once an individual has invested so
much in his personality that he feels he can no longer afford to change
it, he uses crutches to help cope with life's pace. Whenever you use a
crutch you run the risk of becoming dependent upon it.

You can become addicted to almost anything. All addictions are fundamentally identical, even though substances differ in their power to
addict, because people become addicted to thrills. Thrills are due to
chemical changes in the brain. Inspiring music, works of art, Nature's
glories, films, ballets, plays, books, sports events, parades, perfumes,
food, gambling, exercise, sex and everything else which overwhelms
you with tingling excitement give you pleasure because of internal
molecules.

Some researchers believe that thrills occur when molecules called endorphins are released. A drug called naloxone blocks those molecules
and prevents music from inspiring you, movies from stirring you, and
parades from creating a lump in your throat. Other researchers credit
adrenalin and other hormones with thrills, and some like Vimalananda
regarded increased blood flow into certain sections of the brain as the
cause of exaltation. Whatever the specific cause chemistry is at the basis
of thrills and addictions.

Our society is inundated by addictions because we crave intensity
and require ever stronger thrills to satisfy our cravings. Humans who

become addicted to intensity can exhaust their internal thrill molecules, and then may turn to certain foods for stimulation, or may use drugs as substitutes. Addiction to drugs reduces sensitivity to the simpler thrills of life, and weakens our very humanity. Rats administered morphine lose all maternal instinct and refrain from showing maternal behavior to their offspring. Naloxone returns their behavior to normal. Endorphins, which are internally derived opiates, may have a similar effect. We cannot afford to purchase painlessness at the cost of maternal instinct, because we are dependent for health on Nature, the Universal Mother.

Subtlety has gone out of fashion in our society. Our nervous systems are no longer sensitive enough to function at the level of "art, grace and culture" which for Vimalananda distinguishes human beings from animals in human form, those who have lost interest in differentiating between right and wrong.

Animals also self-administer drugs to themselves on occasion. Baboons have been known to use tobacco; elephants, raccoons, bears, goats, pigs and sheep consume fermented fruits and grains for the alcohol; and reindeer, cattle and rabbits sometimes partake of intoxicating mushrooms. Animals know when to stop, though. Once dedicated to intensity humans rarely stop willingly, because unlike animals who use their intoxicants for an occasional change of pace humans use their crutches to balance themselves.

V people usually become addicted to substances which reduce their pain and insecurity. P people adopt addictions which keep them at the high level of activity which they associate with success. K people often fall into addiction unawares because of poor eating habits which they fail to change. Sweet addiction is a good example of how addictions develop.

Sweet creates satisfaction in Ahamkara. If you search for satisfaction primarily in your food instead of in your life, you may become addicted to Sweet. If you are not careful to select healthful Sweet foods like fruit and whole grains you will probably fall prey to sugar-filled junk foods like doughnuts for your Sweet fix. When you eat too much white sugar for too long you become hypersensitive to it. It exhausts your system's ability to digest it and aggravates Vata, which increases with any sort of exhaustion. Vata then exaggerates the gap between your high blood sugar level and your low blood sugar level. The degree of variation between the two is determined by the intensity of your Vata disturbance, and determines in turn the severity of your symptoms. Control of Vata eases the symptoms.

You cannot shake a Sweet addiction by trying to go off it cold turkey onto other tastes. You must first replace refined sugar with other Sweet foods like whole grains so that you still get a Sweet "fix" regularly during the day. Ayurvedic supplements can then be used to even out the "spikiness" in your system's response to carbohydrates which causes the roller-coastering of your blood sugar. Simultaneously, a good diet and good habits will reduce and balance Vata.

Alcohol is a sort of super-Sweet substance, one which is metabolized in the same way as sugar. The tremendous Sweet rush which alcohol gives gratifies Ahamkara tremendously. Alcoholics are people who find the alcohol-Sweet so superior to other forms of Sweet that they insist on prolonging their experience of it. Alcohol is a medicine in small amounts, but overuse makes it a poison. When you ingest alcohol regularly your system creates a balance for itself based on alcohol, and you eventually begin to feel ill if you fail to drink regularly. You are addicted, even if you are not a classic alcoholic.

Any habit which you cannot break without seriously damaging your body, mind or spirit persona is an addiction. All addictions must be broken, though it is usually best to break them gradually so that the system does not go dramatically out of balance in the process. Each addiction requires special consideration. Because alcohol abuse is so common, some elements of the Ayurvedic approach to alcohol dependency are presented here.

Alcohol dependency is a form of Sweet dependency in which all three Doshas are disturbed. Small amounts of medicinal wines control Vata-type diseases; larger amounts of alcohol cause Vata diseases. Alcohol, because of its hot, intense taste and smell and its liquid nature, aggravates both Pitta and Kapha, which then create obstructions to the free movement of Vata and vitiate it. The late stages of alcoholism are purely Vata in nature: shuffling gait, vacant stare, profuse and meaningless speech, severe mood swings, delirium tremens, and hallucinations. All these symptoms reflect profound mental and physical "jerkiness" as a result of the erraticalness of deranged Vata. Even if you are not frankly alcoholic, you will have to calm Vata first and then bring Kapha and Pitta back to normal if you want to eliminate an alcohol habit.

Modern medicine has determined that there is a definite genetic sensitivity to alcohol which is present in 7 to 10% of the population. In other words the tendency to alcoholism is passed from parent to child genetically. There seem to be two types of genetic alcohol sensitivity. The first, which need not be too severe, can be passed from father or mother to son or daughter and usually causes alcoholism to develop only after age 25. The second type is passed only from father to son. The affected individual can be shown to have significant inherited brain abnormalities even if he never drinks, but most victims begin drinking as early as age 11 or 12 and become alcoholic quickly. Unlike the first type, their behavior is often violent.

People who have been dependent on alcohol and then give it up often trade their addiction to alcohol for addictions to coffee, into which they may pour heaps of sugar, and to Hot, Sour, Salty, Pungent food, like French fries with ketchup and chili sauce. Coffee and chili sauce, both Pungent, replace that aspect of alcohol's Taste personality. Intensive use of white sugar is the easiest way for the body to get the level of Sweet intake which alcohol has made it accustomed to. Ketchup and other sauces provide the necessary levels of Sour and Salty to force the already overburdened digestive tract sufficiently to handle the heavy, fried food, whose heaviness and oil help reduce Vata. Each of these Tastes must be provided to the alcoholic body to permit it to preserve its relative balance. The Bitter Taste is used simultaneously to reduce the organism's intensity requirements.

Sweet should be provided by whole grains, and by fruits and fruit juices. Grains provide a regular, stable source of sugar to the blood, and fruit juices like grape or pear should be used to provide quick "fixes" of Sweet when the body demands them. Pomegranate juice provides Sweet along with Astringency, which is further therapeutic for Pitta. Dates are good sources of Sweet because they strengthen the body.

Carrot juice is Hot enough to encourage good digestion, and Bitter enough to help reduce the body's need for intense stimulation. It is also powerfully Sweet. The satisfaction and balance which the body receives from carrot juice provides tremendous subliminal satisfaction to the brain, which compensates to some extent for the lack of pleasurable mental distortion alcohol can provide.

Carrot juice may be consumed alone. If the liver is especially deranged beet can be added. Adding the long white daikon radish helps support weak digestion. Cucumber's Astringency helps reduce intensity craving and soothe inflamed tissues. The best addition is cilantro, which is Pungent but Cold. It is one of the best foods available for reducing anger, as it flushes heat from both body and mind. If the digestion is very weak, radish and carrot can be pressure-cooked together with a slice of beet into a soup, or these vegetables can be chopped and cooked with mung beans and rice into kichadi, and cilantro added on top.

Fresh coconut milk is an excellent Sweet unless liver weakness forces a restricted fat intake. It is usually available bottled in health food stores. Otherwise the flesh of a fresh coconut should be shredded, put into a blender, and covered with just enough water to wet all of it. After blending it should be strained, more cold water should be added, and the process repeated. Hot water should then be added, and after this straining the remains of the coconut meat should be discarded. Coconut is cooling, and heavy for digestion; its heaviness helps satisfy the alcoholic's craving for heavy food.

Lemon or lime juice should provide the Sour Taste in the diet, and the Salty Taste should be provided with kelp or other seaweed powder, or with a liquid-amino preparation. The Amalaki fruit if available is the best source of Sourness. Dry ginger is the best source of Pungency, but it should be used carefully to prevent further Pitta disturbance.

Mild laxation is good purification for someone who has abused alcohol since it eliminates accumulated heat from the liver which is afflicted by increased Pitta. Bitter can be provided by the compounds Arogya Vardhini and Tikta, or by a variety of single herbs including gentian, barberry and aloe vera, all of which also flush toxins from the liver. Dramatic purgation should be avoided because although it quickly reduces Pitta it will further aggravate Vata by its intensity. Since a craving for intensity is one aspect of dependence on alcohol or other drugs, reduction of the organism's exposure to intensity is therapeutic.

Physiological balancing removes jerkiness and promotes stability, which in turn assists the mind to right itself and return to normal functioning. People drink alcohol because it inflates Ahamkara past her boundaries. These people exist in pure Ahamkara energy, pure individuality, without regard for spirit, mind, or body. The self-disgust and self-pity an alcoholic shows when he or she is sober is a trick that Ahamkara plays on the rest of the organism so that it can continue uninterruptedly enjoying its alcohol-food. Alcoholism is, in fact, a disease of Ahamkara, of the individuality.

Alcohol is a super-Sweet. No ordinary food can match the intense current of Sweetness which flows with alcohol into the brain. To partially substitute, flood all the senses with Sweet. Let the patient's nose smell Sweet fragrances, like rose, and let his skin feel "Sweet" things, like oil. "Sweet words" should fall into the patient's ears, and "Sweet" surroundings, like life in the country, should meet his eyes. Intense Sweet of all sorts must be provided until the brain is willing and able to scale down its Sweet intake. Otherwise the patient may backslide and return to alcohol, which he or she knows can be relied on to provide Sweetness.

The mind must be strengthened if its faculty of discrimination is to reassert itself. Memory and discrimination can both be strengthened with the herb gotu kola, taken as a tea or in capsules washed down with tea of the herb skullcap. Gotu kola is the main ingredient in the Ayurvedic medicine Brahmi Vati.

An alcoholic's worst mental problem is weakness of will. The alcohol-dependent Ahamkara believes she can live without body, mind, or spirit, and is willing to deceive body, mind and spirit as long as she can. To perpetuate her unrestricted indulgence she weakens the individual will-power until it can no longer object to her desire to drink. Nothing can be done to remedy this addiction until the individual will-power reasserts itself and reestablishes limits for Ahamkara. As my teacher Vimalananda put it, "If you want to drink, you must make sure that you are drinking the drink, and that the drink is not drinking you." The alcohol-dependent Ahamkara allows drink to consume her whole organism, in return for the false promise of eternal life and vitality that the intoxication of alcohol provides.

Ayurveda recognized alcoholism to be a grave disease more than 3,000 years ago, respecting it for its puissance and its potential to cause harm, and insisting that an alcohol-dependent individual accept outside help to put Ahamkara back in her place. This same sort of going outside oneself to seek help is used by modern-day programs which recognize that the first step in management of any dependency is the recognition that a problem exists. Recognition that Ahamkara has gone beyond her limits opens the door to a new balance for the entire organism.

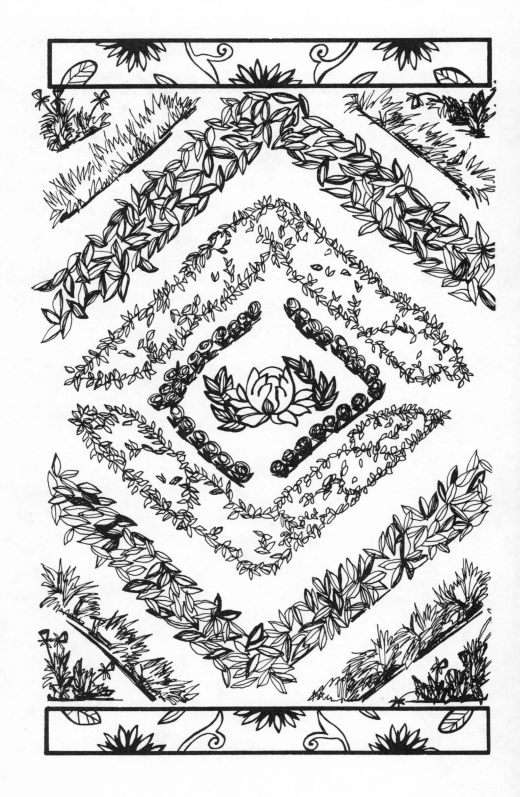

Chapter Four

Nutrition

The Seven Dhatus

Digested food nourishes both body and mind, and provides strength and support for Ahamkara and her beloved personality. Ayurveda divides all body tissues into seven classes called Dhatus, a Dhatu being anything which provides firmness. Each Dhatu satisfies one of the Ahamkara's requirements for existence in a human body, and "firms up" or "confirms" Ahamkara's self-identity with the body. How well you—your personality—fits in your body will determine your resistance to the aliens who challenge your claim to your organism.

The Seven Dhatus are:

Rasa - literally, "sap" or "juice"; tissue fluids, including chyle, lymph, and blood plasma. Its accessory tissues are breast milk and menstrual blood, and its waste product is mucus. Its function is Prinana, or nourishment.

Blood - red blood cells. Its accessory tissues are blood vessels and tendons, and its waste is bile. Its function is Jivana, or invigoration.

Flesh - skeletal muscle. Its accessory tissues are ligaments and skin, and its wastes are those which accumulate in body orifices: ear wax, snot, navel lint, smegma, and so on. Its function is Lepana, or "plastering" of the skeleton.

Fat - fat in the limbs and torso. Its accessory tissue is omentum, and its waste is sweat. Snehana, or lubrication, is its function.

Bone - all bones. Its accessories are the teeth, and its wastes body hair, beard, and nails. It provides the body Dharana, or support.

Marrow - anything inside a bone: red and yellow bone marrow, and the brain and spinal cord, which are wholly encased in bone. Its accessory tissue is head hair, and lachrymal secretions are its wastes. It performs Purana, or "filling" of the bones.

Shukra - male and female sexual fluids. Its tasks are Garbhotpatti, or reproduction, and production of Ojas, the fluid which produces the aura and controls immunity. It has neither accessory tissues nor waste products.

This scheme is not a fully detailed explanation of human physiology. The Rishis were not interested in minute detail; they looked deeper, trying to discover organizing principles. This is an explanation of how Ahamkara chooses to clothe herself in flesh.

As long as the Dhatus are healthy and well-formed, and the wastes are minimal and quickly excreted, Ahamkara experiences maximal satisfaction in her incarnation and the individual experiences a deep somatic sense of well-being. When there is inadequate Dhatu nutrition Ahamkara feels this lack, and her dissatisfaction is transmitted to the consciousness of the individual in question. Digestion and assimilation are essential to an individual's well-being at all levels.

Ayurveda states that each Dhatu is formed from the one immediately previous to it, except the accessory tissues, which are only nourished and do not nourish in return. Breast milk and endometrium, for example, are meant for nourishing a child and play no further part in the mother's nutrition. The wastes produced at each stage of Dhatu digestion are used in diagnosis, because excess of any waste is indicative of poor digestion at the level of that Dhatu.

Most of us would readily accept that ingested food first forms chyle, which then produces red blood cells, which then go to nourish flesh. There our common-sense understanding of the process ceases, though. How can flesh nourish fat, or bone nourish marrow? The answer lies in a re-definition of the word "nourish." These Dhatus "nourish" one another by providing metabolic conditions which are conducive to production of the next in line, and by each satisfying a need of Ahamkara which allows the next need to be addressed.

For example, if Bone is metabolically unhealthy, the body's chemical environment becomes less conducive to proper formation of Marrow, which then is less able to form healthy Shukra. The texts recognize three ways in which this environment can be influenced:

1. One Dhatu may completely convert itself into another. For example, Rasa provides direct nourishment for the production of Blood. A large part of circulating Rasa is converted into Blood. The Ayurvedic analogy is to the formation of yogurt from milk.

2. The Dhatu may flow through the body, gradually nourishing the next Dhatu in line through a more complicated series of reactions. For example, when Blood nourishes Flesh it flows through many different parts of the body, nourishing Flesh all along the line. The traditional analogy was to the flow of irrigation water through a ditch in a field.

3. The Dhatu may merely "seed" the next Dhatu, by sending hor-

monal or enzymatic cues to it. This is the way Flesh nourishes Fat and Fat nourishes Bone. It is compared in Ayurveda to the random seeding of a field by a pigeon dropping seeds from its beak.

RASA DHATU

Ahamkara and the Dhatus are mutually interdependent. Without Ahamkara's OK no molecule can be admitted into the fellowship of your body; without well-nourished Dhatus Ahamkara's confidence, which controls its ability to maintain the body's immune defenses, is impaired. Either way health suffers.

The progression of the Seven Dhatus represents the seven stages involved in Ahamkara's nourishment. This integration of external, alien material into your internal being is a sensitive operation which begins with the introduction of food into your mouth. Tastes alert the brain to the sort of food which has been ingested; the brain directs the digestive process accordingly. As digestion proceeds, material which has undergone preliminary conversion is absorbed into the system and begins to circulate. This Dhatu is Rasa.

Rasa has at least two dozen important meanings in Sanskrit, meanings as varied as water, semen, plant sap, and metallic mercury. Rasa Dhatu mainly signifies chyle, blood plasma and lymph, but it also refers to "taste" and "emotion." The fact that Rasa means "taste" indicates that good Rasa Dhatu can be produced only when the ingested food possesses the Tastes required by the organism. Those Tastes ensure that the Doshas do their jobs properly.

Vata, Pitta and Kapha in turn determine how efficiently digestion and assimilation can occur. Vata controls the movement of nutrients to the cells and wastes from the cells. Insufficient nutrients or excessive wastes interfere with Dhatu nutrition. Kapha provides the structures in which these movements occur; disturbed structures mean disturbed transport. Pitta is in charge of conversion of nutrient into body part, and determines how much nutrient will be used and how much waste will be produced.

Rasa Dhatu's special function is "Prinana," a word which means nourishment but is derived from a root which signifies romantic love. All bodies live from meal to meal, eternally craving further food. When the body is hungry, each of its cells is hungry. Just as a plant who is withering from lack of attention and water seems to freshen immediately when sprinkled by a thoughtful passerby, so too all of your cells perk up, physically and emotionally, when they receive the "sap" of Rasa Dhatu. Rasa is not sufficient in itself to nourish the whole organism, but it is a promise of better things to come.

Romance is an ephemeral emotion, which projects a potential to provide more. Likewise, the satisfaction you feel from a glass of juice at the end of a long fast, or the relief your organism experiences when you drink a glass of water after several hours of thirst, is really just an anticipation of the nourishment your tissues will experience after your digestion operates on the food or water. "Prinana" is the satisfaction you feel when the nourishment first enters your system.

It is called "romantic love" because it is really a waltz of two separate existences—you and the food—who are trying to become sufficiently intimate with one another to unite together. The sense of danger, the exaltation of excitement, the thrill of the unknown, and all the other emotions including the lust you feel when you fall in love you also feel, in simpler form, when your body is suffused with the fresh Rasa from a well-digested meal.

If your food is not properly digested, or if it is well-digested but improperly assimilated, your Ahamkara will feel precisely like the lover whose date stands her up: cheated, used, abused and frustrated. To be led on (by the process of digestion after thorough chewing and swallowing) to expect a night on the town (good assimilation of healthy Rasa), and then to wait for hours in growing despair as your corsage wilts, is an affront to self-confidence (a weakening of Ahamkara's power to project a unified personality), and can lead to self-denigration (weakening of immunity) if it happens frequently.

The texts list many symptoms which develop when Rasa is disturbed. The most important are "lack of faith," and "lack of taste." "Lack of faith" develops from lack of self-confidence. It shows a lack of faith in yourself, in others, or both, depending on whether your Ahamkara concludes that its failure to be nourished derived from its own insufficiency or from the malicious intervention of some outside party. Lack of faith can develop into suspicion, and suspicion can create barriers against whatever aspect of the outside or inside world has been adjudged by Ahamkara to be guilty of treachery.

"Lack of taste" has a twin meaning. Physiologically it indicates a lack of desire for food, which happens when Ama is produced in preference to Rasa. The system then recognizes that it must first digest Ama, to clear the obstruction to the Dhatu nourishment process, before any further nutrition is taken in.

Psychologically, "lack of taste" means lack of interest in living, "lack of flavor for the things in life." Unable to get excited about anything, the afflicted individual moves about in a perpetual funk. This is a form of lovesickness: bereft of the love object, the lover moves about in a fog, unable to derive satisfaction from normal pursuits. Here the lover is Ahamkara and the love object is Rasa. The funk is Kapha, the waste product produced at the stage of conversion of food into Rasa. Inefficient conversion produces excessive Kapha, which encourages Ama production and creates this lethargy.

If Ahamkara's suitor (the food) is exposed to be a criminal (Ama), a being who actually wishes her harm, he must be kicked out of the house and out of the relationship. Ahamkara must then repair her broken heart, turn her back on her previous life (avoid certain foods and undergo therapeutic procedures) and wait patiently for a new suitor. No personality can be mentally and emotionally healthy until its physical body is freed of indigestion.

BLOOD

When your organism is able to obtain sufficient Rasa, the date between your Ahamkara and her nourishment takes place, and Rasa has a chance to be converted into Blood. Blood produces "invigoration," that rush of vitality which makes us feel the full vibrancy of life. Some of the sense of danger evaporates as the Ahamkara gets to know her date and finds him exciting and stimulating. He has "got into her blood." She is fascinated by him; she begins to think that maybe he is a fit mate for her. Hope and anticipation invigorate her.

When Rasa is not well digested Blood is insufficiently produced and Pitta, the waste product at this stage, is overproduced. Pitta is a hot, intense influence, just like Blood, but Pitta cannot perform Blood's function of invigoration. Pitta can only heat up the organism, resulting in increased anger (at the love object for refusing to submit to domination by Ahamkara) and jealousy (lest any other Ahamkara dare to try to snatch the roving love object away). "Hot-blooded lovers" have ample Rasa for romance or lust, but they have too much Pitta in their blood; their violence is a manifestation of this heat energy as it exits after scorching the individual.

FLESH

When Blood is healthy and well-formed it nourishes Flesh, whose job is "plastering," covering of the skeleton and internal organs so that they are not exposed to the outside. The wastes produced at this stage are wastes which develop in and occlude body orifices. Flesh also provides a preliminary barrier between the "you" of your organism and the "not-you" of the external world. Your muscle fibers are like bricks and stones in your body's fortifications against attack from without; they provide a sense of security.

To continue with our analogy of the date, our couple—the Ahamkara and her food—have decided to go steady. He will now defend her as his against all challenges; she now has a protector, a "bodyguard," to shelter her from the world. An Ahamkara who lacks sufficient healthy Flesh feels naked and defenseless, uncovered to the world, open to external influences in spite of romance and invigoration. Body builders who turn away from all other human pursuits in order to magnify their muscles are often insecure individuals who use those muscles to insulate themselves from the need to interact substantively with anyone on the outside.

FAT

Well-nourished Flesh feeds Fat, whose function is "Sneha," which literally means unctuousness. Sneha also means love, though it is love of a different sort from Prinana. Sneha is a bonded, secure love relationship, like that which exists between mother and child, or husband and wife. Just as loving partners snuggle and cuddle together for warmth, fat "snuggles" our bodies and provides us warm, satisfying love. Ahamkara and her food have finally tied the knot; they are now wed to one another, for better or for worse. Fat, and to some extent Flesh as well, provide us with that sublime satisfaction that a sound sleeper receives from a warm quilt on a cold night.

Fat and its waste product sweat both help maintain the body's internal temperature. Fat insulates us to hold heat in; sweat radiates heat away. A human whose Fat is insufficient is perpetually physically and emotionally cold, lacking that thermal insulation which Fat provides. This coldness makes the individual seek increased physical and mental nourishment, without much concern for the means used, to nourish Fat and achieve the warm, satisfying love it can give. Remember Cassius and his "lean and hungry look." Cassius searched for gratification, not for love, as does anyone who enjoys lust, invigoration and physical security while assiduously avoiding sincere emotional commitment. It is possible that the anorexic look which is so popular in fashion today is partly derived from the drive for independence and rootlessness which breaks bonds and restrictive relationships and displays itself psychosomatically as a near-pathological aversion to Fat.

Extreme overabundance of Fat is characteristic of those people who despair of locating a bonded love relationship with another human and turn to the solace that Fat can provide. Such warm-hearted people simply lack that loving life-partner or that stable family situation which could act as an object for the affection. The satisfaction an obese individual feels in being fat is real and perceptible to Ahamkara, and the likelihood of successful, permanent weight loss is low until Ahamkara is redirected and becomes willing to relinquish the "security blanket" to which she clings. This affection must be directed at other objects, perhaps externally to community service activities, or internally to spiritual development. Obesity is neither a simple psychological problem nor a simple problem of nutrition. It is a problem of psychological nutrition.

BONE

Healthy Fat makes for healthy Bone, whose job is "support." Bone makes it possible for us to move in the world. Without our bony skeletons we would all lie limply in puddles on the floor like jellyfish. The bones and joints are closely connected with the mind's ability to express itself, because capability for expression is a function of ability to move. Bone is "supportive" as well as "supporting"; it allows us to project our own identities out into the world, just as its wastes—body hair, beard and nails—grow and project themselves from the interior out into the exterior. When support is lacking, gratification, invigoration, security and commitment provide only limited satisfaction.

The previous four Dhatus are concerned solely with our internal health and are quite external to our most vital body organs. Bone marks a shift in emphasis. Now the food begins to flow deeply into the organism's interior, into its center, to assist in maintaining external health. Ahamkara's ability to maintain her internal integrity has been protected; now her ability to maintain her external integrity, her ability to present a coherent, unified face to the world, must be stabilized. Weak Bone reduces Ahamkara's support for her external projection. Think of the epithet "spineless wonder" and you have a mental picture of the effect of unhealthy Bone on an individual. Healthy Bone allows Ahamkara to concrete her personality and establish firm personal parameters.

MARROW

Bone produces Marrow. Marrow is anything inside a bone, including the fatty yellow bone marrow, the blood-forming red bone marrow, and the brain and spinal cord, which are entirely encased in Bone. Note that although Marrow physically produces Blood, Blood is identified in Ayurveda with the liver, which modern medicine knows to be the controller of blood production, if not its actual site. Ayurveda is interested in root causes.

The function of Marrow is "filling." Physiologically, Bone is as prone to accumulation of Vata as the colon is, because both are hollow; this is one reason for their mutual affinity. The "filling" of Marrow discourages Vata accumulation. On the mental plane, healthy Marrow prevents emptiness of mind. Already the food has provided the Ahamkara a firm foundation against which to brace while projecting; any good spouse would do this. Now the food dives deeper into the depths of the organism and pools itself inside the Bony bastions which Ahamkara has created for it. As Marrow it acts as an energy-storage medium, something like a computer memory bank: a pool of passive, available power.

The mere ability to project your personality into the world is insufficient. You may feel gratified, invigorated, secure, loved and confident, but unless there is something of value present in your personality which can be projected, you are hollow, your "headpiece filled with straw," your words "full of sound and fury and signifying nothing." This is a very prevalent disease today, and is characteristic of the world's generally poor state of nutrition. It is diagnosable from the eyes, which are the single most significant projector of the personality into the environment.

Healthy Marrow gives the eyes a clear, strong sheen which radiates calm light just like a lamp flame in a quiet place; dull, lifeless eyes are indicative of weak Marrow. In some terminal diseases, like galloping consumption, the eyes become feverishly bright toward the end. This does not indicate health, of course; it shows that the organism has marshalled its last fading reserves of strength and is using them to project its personality outwards for as long as it has left. The body burns its own tissues to provide light to project its Ahamkara through its windows on the world, the eyes.

Because Bone is one of the chief seats of Vata, and because Marrow is derived from Bone, Marrow is prone to inadequate nutrition, even if the rest of the body is healthy, because of the drying, roughening and destabilizing effects of Vata. Weak Marrow will not directly affect Bone's nutrition adversely, though it can do so indirectly. Some empty-Marrow individuals can project their personalities into the world and influence others with great ease. They are forceful and persuasive, but there is no substance to their projection. It is all so much "hot air," being a product of Vata. This Vata disturbance eventually affects Bone, which is so prone to Vata derangement. When the bloated balloon of the inflated, aggrandized personality finally bursts, all the air whooshes out and the individual is left crumpled in a heap on the ground.

SHUKRA AND OJAS

Properly nourished Marrow goes to nourish Shukra, the collective word for all secretions involved in reproduction. The food has now been transformed into a substance which can unite with Ahamkara. Shukra's functions are creation and creativity. Shukra can be used for procreation, which is the production of children, or it can be used for the production of artistic or intellectual creations. Shukra's job is to act as a matrix through which new creations can manifest on our plane of existence. It is the clay which creativity shapes into forms.

Weak Shukra means weak creativity. Afflicted individuals may have it all; they may be gratified, invigorated, secure and loved, may be able to project themselves cogently and coherently into their environment, and may have plenty to offer, but without strong Shukra they will be unable to consummate any productive arrangement or exert any lasting effect on the flow of events. A child is a lasting effect; so is a new corporation, a sheaf of music, or an amended law. Shukra controls an individual's ability to make a mark on the slate of the world.

When Ahamkara couples excitedly and expansively with Shukra the energy aroused becomes uncontrollable. It then flows out of the body into another body via the sex act, or into some project or enterprise. When the Ahamkara couples with Shukra calmly and collectedly, the new substance created remains within the body and solidifies the link between the physical, mental and spiritual existences. This substance is called Ojas.

All forms of physical and mental indigestion damage Ojas and encourage Ama formation. Indigestion is easiest to deal with when it is limited to the digestive tract. Once it moves into the Dhatus, and disrupts the Ahamkara's ability to nourish herself, its management becomes much more complicated. If Ama blocks Dhatu nutrition in your digestive tract, your life first loses its zest as Rasa becomes malnourished and polluted with Kapha. Then Pitta-polluted Blood saps your vitality, malnourished Flesh strips you of your security, and each Dhatu in turn is weakened until Ojas, the foundation of your immunity, is starved into dysfunction. Mind pollutes body by forcing it into unhealthy activities, and body pollutes mind by producing Ama and starving the organism of Ojas. Mind and body are concurrently and inherently joined.

Obesity

Because so many people in the world have more Fat than they need obesity is an appropiate illustration of the interaction between mind and body and its implications for the Dhatus and for Ahamkara. Obesity, like gout and diabetes, is classified in Ayurveda as one of the "diseases of affluence." Affluence is not restricted to the rich; every one of us who has time or money to waste is affluent. Affluence, or rather the affluent state of mind which believes it has time and money to waste, is the real disease; obesity, gout and diabetes are only its symptoms.

Most residents of the affluent countries of the West feel "affluent," and it is not surprising that most of us Westerners need to lose some weight. This is why our popular culture worships thinness, and why the incidence of anorexia is so high. Other cultures, like that of India, have an entirely different concept of beauty than do we. No one in India, no matter how wealthy, believes that thin is beautiful. Every hero and heroine of the Indian silver screen is plump. The incidence of anorexia in India and in other developing countries is negligible because people there enjoy the Ahamkara-gratification which Fat provides.

Our culture prizes individuality over bonding to society, and so the bonding which the Fat Dhatu provides is not valued highly. However, at the same time mass advertising exhorts us to consume continuously, since constant consumption is the mechanism by which our affluence has been obtained. An Ayurvedic text comments: "Boredom, mindless entertainment, continuous eating, and oversleeping: these will fatten you up just like a hog." Most of us have experienced the truth of this saying during holidays when liberated from drudgery we stuff ourselves like pigs and then watch TV until we become so bored and indolent that we fall asleep. This is an infallible way to gain weight, and if repeated regularly it can lead to obesity.

We are bombarded daily with conflicting suggestions: eat constantly and feel affluent, but never gain weight! It is a wonder that more of us have not been driven insane by such incongruous suggestions. Many of

us who have not lost our senses from this incongruity have become neu-
rotic, though, and neurosis is enough to cause a person to become obese.
Food neuroses develop from the suppression of these conflicting emotions, and from the influence of internal chemical imbalances. Internal
confusion encourages us to recede further into affluence, which compounds the problem. The causes of obesity are so entwined with one
another that it is impossible to separate the excess weight and the
emotional trauma. Any approach to weight loss must consider all causes.

Some people are better able than others to satisfy the paradoxical
cultural requirements of our society. Variations in ability to lose weight
occur because of what modern scientists call the "fat setpoint," the level
of fat your body tries to maintain because it functions best at that level.
The main influence on this "fat setpoint" is your genetics acting through
your personal constitution. V people burn food quickly and have to intensively overeat in order to become obese. VP people are almost this
lucky, and P people can usually lose any weight they might temporarily
gain. VK people are slow to gain weight and equally slow to lose it. PK
and K people always seem to have some extra poundage somewhere
that they want to get rid of no matter how little they eat.

Another critical influence occurs during infancy when the number of
fat cells you have is finalized. These fat cells once formed are permanent
residents of your body; when you lose weight the amount of fat within
each one is reduced but they themselves never disappear. Children who
are overfed poor diets are sure to develop a large number of fat cells
and until the ends of their lives will find it easy to gain weight and difficult to take it off again. Fat babies make for fat adults.

Attitude also counts. Fear tends to refuse to allow nutrients into the
system, which is why V people often have difficulty gaining weight.
However, anyone who overeats to calm fear will eventually gain weight.
Anger burns away nutrients, which is how P people may escape obesity despite their strong hunger, but anyone who overeats specifically to
cool anger eventually gains weight. K people tend to hold weight on
anyway, and anyone who overeats to gratify a need for Fat-type bonded
love (a Kapha-mediated reason) is sure to gain weight. People who,
filled with Bitterness due to intense frustration, choose to obtains life's
Sweetness through food may become addicted to the pleasures of eating and may become obese. Individual reasons for obesity vary, but all
of them involve the determination of Ahamkara to hold tenaciously to
her beloved Fat, the Dhatu which provides reliable, steady love and
warmth.

No diet, however strict, can change this. Loneliness is worse for you
than a high-fat diet when you are trying to lose weight. Most strict diets
are actually self-defeating because they manifest from an attitude of self-
hatred, of disgust for the fat and for the self whose weakness allowed
the fat to accumulate. This attitude leads to a desire to starve the body

in order to punish the mind. The body feels starved during any crash diet, and because it does not like to be starved it acts on its own to preserve its highest energy tissue by lowering its metabolic rate, which burns fat more slowly. It also tends to first burn off those tissues which are not immediately needed. Anyone who diets but does not exercise will therefore lose lean tissue first since it is not being used.

Hunger pangs increase as the body tries to force the mind to eat more and satisfy its hunger. This affects junk food addicts worst, since their bodies have been emptied of many essential nutrients which their bodies experience severe hunger for when dieting. Moreover, when dieters go back to their normal eating habits at the end of a diet they burn off less calories and store more fat than they did previously, because their metabolic rates have dropped, and because their bodies are now wary of starvation and want to store even more just in case such an episode should be repeated. Crash dieting therefore increases the body's fat setpoint, and makes you fatter!

The psychological effects of crash dieting are even more pernicious. Both starving people and dieters dream and fantasize about food, and both suffer from anxiety and depression, all from the physical stress of having to live below the body's desired fat setpoint. The body and mind of a dieter are at daggers drawn with one another. When the organism cheats on its diet because it can no longer withstand the body's incessant demands for food, the mind's first reaction is to binge, because "I've already gone off my diet, so why not?" After the binge guilt rears up, as the mind realizes that its temporary indulgence in food has damaged its physical self-image. To remedy this the dieter returns to penance and starts back down the road to starvation, little knowing that such erratic behavior inexorably drives up the setpoint, and also aggravates Vata.

Even resisting temptation can be hazardous to your weight. Every dieter who lusts after a luscious dessert sends a message to the brain that new and tasty morsels are about to be consumed. This makes the mouth water and the digestive juices start to flow, and signals the body's insulin to remove some sugar from the general circulation to make way for the new sugar which will soon be flooding the blood. The body stores this sugar as fat.

Lowered blood sugar increases the appetite. Whenever you crave a tempting dessert but restrain yourself from eating it, you add a little fat at the moment of craving, and when you next eat you will eat more than you would normally have eaten because your mental lust for the dessert has lowered your blood sugar and increased both your physical appetite for carbohydrate and your mental appetite for Sweet. Added body fat increases insulin production, which causes more and more fat to be deposited at each episode. You really can gain weight just by looking at a tasty pastry!

Eventually excess fat makes your insulin less sensitive to your blood sugar level, because the body resists laying down any more fat after it passes its preferred setpoint. Then your blood sugar begins to increase above normal, which means diabetes. When the tissues lose their ability to use insulin the muscles feel starved, because they cannot get their regular supply of sugar fuel, and they will send persistent demands to the brain for more food, thus deepening the downward spiral of malnutrition and damaging Ahamkara further. Overnourishment of a Dhatu is as bad or worse than undernourishment.

Most cases of diabetes which develop in this way do not require insulin for treatment, because weight loss can return insulin function to normal and ensure that the tissues are again well fed. Diabetes, like all "diseases of affluence," responds well to austerity.

Losing Weight

Permanent weight loss occurs only when the body's setpoint is lowered. The amphetamines in prescription diet pills and the nicotine in tobacco can temporarily lower the fat setpoint, but these effects last only as long as you use the drug. You are bound to gain weight as soon as stop smoking or quit swallowing the pills. Besides, both amphetamines and nicotine are addictive drugs; nicotine is even more addictive than heroin.

These two drugs lower the body's fat setpoint by speeding up the organism, making both body and brain work faster. Speed of any sort increases Vata, which makes both body and mind crave increased Sweet for balance. Both nicotine and amphetamines provide a certain intense Sweet to the brain but not to the body, and when the drug is removed the accumulated physical craving of the tissues for nutrition forces the individual to eat excessively, leading to guilt at indiscipline, further dramatic attempts to lose weight, and generalized Vata increase, which deepens the neurosis.

Ayurveda believes in speeding up the organism in healthy, natural ways, such as exercise, certain supplements, and the use of light, non-Kapha-producing foods, which control Vata while relieving the system of excess Kapha. It is a slower process, but in weight loss, as in all other aspects of medicine, haste makes waste.

If you are overweight and suffer from all or most of the following symptoms, you urgently need to reduce your poundage under competent professional guidance:

Pendulous belly, breasts, and buttocks; Puffing and panting for breath even on mild exertion; Profuse perspiration even when it is not hot; Excess thirst, especially at night; Intense food craving; Prolonged but unsatisfying sleep; Unpleasant body odor; Inflammation where skin folds rub against one another; Generalized body ache; Loss of sexual appetite; Lack of zeal or enthusiasm for living.

If you do not suffer from most of these symptoms you should not attempt severe dieting or other heroic attempts to lose weight. You may still be benefitted by guidance, however, especially if you have an addiction to food. A few people are strong-willed enough to succeed on their own, but most people require some external source of support when they are trying to relinquish an addiction. It might be a spouse, a close friend, or a group of individuals who all suffer from the same problem, but it must be a source of support in which you can place your complete trust, allowing your actions to be guided as you accept advice on how to proceed. You should be willing to accept any assistance that might be offered.

You cannot be in any hurry if you want to make your weight loss permanent. Your body needs time to readjust itself and lower its fat setpoint, and until that setpoint drops your weight will not. Some things, like the development of children in the womb, simply cannot be rushed. In like manner, you are trying to create an entirely new you. A new body silhouette and a new outlook on life require profound personality alterations, and slow progress permits your mind to adjust itself to the new persona. Besides, quick weight loss stresses the body because toxins like DDT which are trapped in the fat are liberated faster than the body's waste disposal systems can handle them. It also stresses Ahamkara, who becomes alarmed when the security of Fat is eliminated before other sources of secure, bonded love can be developed.

Affluence of mind is the true cause of obesity. Your transformation begins when you desist from the boredom which causes you to eat because you feel you have nothing better to do. Being so disgusted with yourself that you eat from sorrow at your seeming inability to change is also a form of affluence. Your goal should be to transform yourself, not to lose weight. Reducing your weight is a part of self-transformation which occurs automatically.

Spring is the best time to begin your bodily renovation, because everything is renewed in spring, and because the warmth of spring and the heat of summer help melt away fat and reset the setpoint. Any time is a good time to begin, though, even if it is beginning again. You should never give up. Even if you fail 100 times, begin again the 101st. Every attempt will benefit you, if it is sincere, and eventually you are bound to succeed.

There is no permanent weight loss without regular exercise. People who exercise four or five times a week lose weight three times faster than those who exercise only thrice a week. Exercise once or twice a week is insufficient to alter the setpoint. Moderate, sustained exercise is better than vigorous exertion. Even a brisk walk for half an hour is sufficient, if it is brisk enough. Strenuous massage acts as a passive exercise which moves the muscles and releases the endorphins. However it suits you, you must get your body moving.

Your breath is especially important. You receive Prana,the life force, from both air and food. Your system will feel less hunger if your breathing is good because it can rely less on food for its Prana. Whenever you feel hungry you should first sit down and take ten deep breaths. If you are still hungry afterwards you can eat, but most of the time you will find that your hunger has faded.

Oversleeping is an important cause of overweight. To reduce your sleep, go to bed each night at the same time and wake up each morning at the same time. If you go to sleep earlier than usual one day you must arise earlier than usual the next morning. Try to arise half and hour before dawn, or at least by 6 a.m. After a month of regularizing your sleep pattern, reduce your total period of sleep by half an hour. Most people find it easiest to go to sleep a half-hour later each night than to get up a half-hour earlier each morning. Reduce your sleep half an hour each month until you reach your minimum. Six hours is good; no one should sleep longer than eight hours except during illness.

If you find you simply cannot reduce your sleep by these means, wake yourself in the middle of the night and get out of bed. Walk around, sit and read, do anything except eat. Stay awake for at least half an hour, and then return to sleep. This breaking up of the soundness of your sleep helps reduce your sleep habit without affecting your rest. Never sleep during the day.

Please follow the suggestions made in the chapter on food, and fast once a week according to your prakruti. Also, increase your eating awareness. Much unnecessary eating is done unconsciously. Some people keep a journal, writing down either before or after the meal a list of foods consumed. Others read their menu into a tape recorder. Still others count to three before each mouthful is eaten. Whatever system you adopt, no matter how silly it may seem, make sure that it requires you to be aware of each substance at every meal.

Be sure to chew thoroughly. Chewing releases flavor from food. Fat people are usually addicted to flavor, so thorough chewing results in more satisfaction from less food. Chewing helps satisfy food cravings on its own, and one way to avoid eating when you crave jaw stimulation is to chew beeswax or even sugarless gum. Eat each food article separately, to achieve greater sensory pleasure. Use one-pot meals only if you need them to control Vata. Refrain from daydreaming or fantasizing about food. Remember that lusting after tasty morsels actually adds to your fat. Take a walk, chew your beeswax, or drink some herbal tea when your imagination becomes overactive.

Reward yourself regularly for good behavior. Permit yourself indulgences in other sensory areas when you achieve success at disciplining your food intake. Make sure that your intake of Sweet through your other senses is sufficient to make up for the Sweet which used to come to you through your tongue. Never punish yourself for backsliding. Punishment for failure reduces hope and confidence for eventual success, reinforces guilt, and weakens the new self-image you are trying to create for yourself. Whenever and whatever you eat, enjoy your food!

If you can observe no other restriction, at least do not eat too fast or too often.

All food which increases Kapha tends to increase weight. Likewise, all food which helps control Kapha discourages weight gain. You should especially avoid the following foods:

Beef and pork; butter, cheese, ice cream, sour cream; wheat and wheat products; white sugar and all products containing white sugar; alcoholic beverages; fried foods of any sort; junk food and fast food; all excessively Sour or Salty foods like pickles.

Merely going on an anti-Kapha diet when you want to lose weight may be entirely inappropriate if you are a V person who needs Kapha-promoting food to maintain balance. It would best for you to stabilize your diet first after removing all the objectionable foods above. Unless your Doshas are balanced your Dhatus including Fat will never become healthy.

Change your diet gradually. Do not salt your food at all; if you want the Salty Taste, use "light" salt, kelp powder, or liquid amino-acid mixtures. Limit your use of sweeteners, but allow yourself regular use of honey, except in cooking. Honey has a mild fat-reducing effect. Take bran or psyllium seed husk whenever you eat a lot of Sweet; fiber helps the body balance its response to Sweet. Even though fruits are Sweet, their fiber usually does not permit their sugars to be absorbed too quickly. The fiber in whole grains also protects against exaggerated blood sugar levels.

Carbohydrates like grains also increase brain serotonin, a chemical which makes you feel relaxed and "mellow." So, even though a high-protein diet may make you lose weight faster, you will lose it more enjoyably and in a more relaxed fashion if you eat a reasonable amount of carbohydrate. Also, fat requires carbohydrate to burn, so trying to deny yourself all carbohydrate while you live on protein and vegetables makes the weight loss more difficult and less certain.

As you feel it is safe and sensible to do so, reduce the quantity of food you eat at each meal. As you reduce your food quantity your stomach will shrink little by little and you will find your capacity for food reduced. Excessive eating is often more a problem with overweight V and P types than it is with overweight Ks, whose bodies tend to hang on to excess pounds even if they do not overeat.

Eliminate all cold food and drink. You should eat nothing that is refrigerator cold. Fat is the body's insulation and increases naturally in colder climates. Continuous exposure to cold food and drink, and even to air conditioning, convinces the body that it should add extra insulation, so up goes the fat setpoint. Exercise, which helps heat the body, reduces its need for insulation.

Reduce your overall water intake as you reduce the salt in your diet. You should drink when you are thirsty, but you do not necessarily need the 6 to 8 glasses of water daily which some "authorities" advocate. Warm water or hot herbal teas help melt fat away. Even better is honey and lemon in warm water, with a pinch of black pepper powder.

When you are fed up with all these restrictions, go out and binge without guilt, preferably on healthful foods, and then forget about it. Cravings for your old food friends are only panic reactions of your body or mind. If you reassure yourself with familiar food that you are not trying to starve to death, the craving to binge will become less and less frequent.

It is wise to take vitamin and mineral supplements during this period of transition to ensure that your body does not lack any nutrients. These supplements cannot reduce your fat setpoint, although Ayurvedic herbal preparations can. These preparations mobilize fat from deposits and eliminate it. These are not appetite suppressants; they are substances which encourage permanent metabolic change so that dietary control and exercise can make the excess fat swiftly disappear and stay away once it is gone.

Any Bitter, Pungent or Astringent food, herb or mineral will exert some weight-reducing effect, though some are more active than others. A few active herbs are barberry, black pepper, gentian, golden seal, gotu kola, red raspberry leaves, saffron, and turmeric. Some Ayurvedic compounds which are prescribed in India for weight reduction include:

The powder called *Triphala*, a mixture of three fruits, especially when mixed with Trikatu, a mixture of equal parts of powdered ginger, black pepper, and Pippali, or long pepper.

The liver purifier *Arogya Vardhini*.

Chandra Prabha, a compound which includes a form of mineral pitch called *Shilajit*.

Guggulu, a gum closely related to myrrh. Guggulu has been used successfully in India to treat such diseases as hepatitis and myocardial necrosis. It helps reduce blood cholesterol, is an emmenagogue and analgesic, and seems to show some anti-fertility activity. The Guggulu formula most used to reduce fat is *Triphala Guggulu*.

Triphala Guggulu's ingredients are Triphala, Trikatu, and Guggulu.

This mixture is then mixed with strong Triphala tea and is rubbed until dry in a mortar and pestle, and small pills are made. Triphala purifies the body of old Ama trapped in the Fat; Trikatu helps lower the body's fat setpoint; and Guggulu actually "scrapes" Fat away from the other tissues. Triphala Guggulu should be taken with warm water or tea of dry ginger.

Many Americans have the notion that if one pill works well, ten should work ten times as well. This is quite untrue. Continued use of larger than normal doses of Guggulu over many months can cause Doshas to accumulate in the lungs and liver. Overuse of Guggulu can aggravate dryness of mouth or body, impotence, darkness of vision, emaciation, faintness, and looseness of the limbs. Fortunately the spice saffron can alleviate Guggulu-caused symptoms. The same precautions apply to the use of myrrh. These side-effects occur only when the system becomes addicted to the presence of Guggulu and is not due to any toxicity on Guggulu's part.

All Ayurvedic preparations work better once you have purified your system. In addition to traditional Ayurvedic purifications it is good to use castor oil before you begin your use of Guggulu. If you are at least 40 pounds heavier than your ideal weight you may for six weeks take 1 Tbsp. of castor oil each morning after arising and wash it down with a strong cup of tea of dry ginger. This will not produce a laxative effect, but will start the scraping action on Fat. You may also use a gland-balancing compound like Tikta for at least a month before beginning with Triphala Guggulu to enhance its effect.

An ideal weight for you is one which is appropriate for your constitution. K types should not try for the anorexic magazine model look. Even though Ayurveda states that it is better to be too thin than too fat, remember that insufficient Fat weakens Ahamkara and damages your immunity. Fat is an essential Dhatu and is good for you, in the proper amount. Hatred of Fat is self-hatred, which gets transferred to Ahamkara and weakens her further. Forget about Fat; think about recreating yourself.

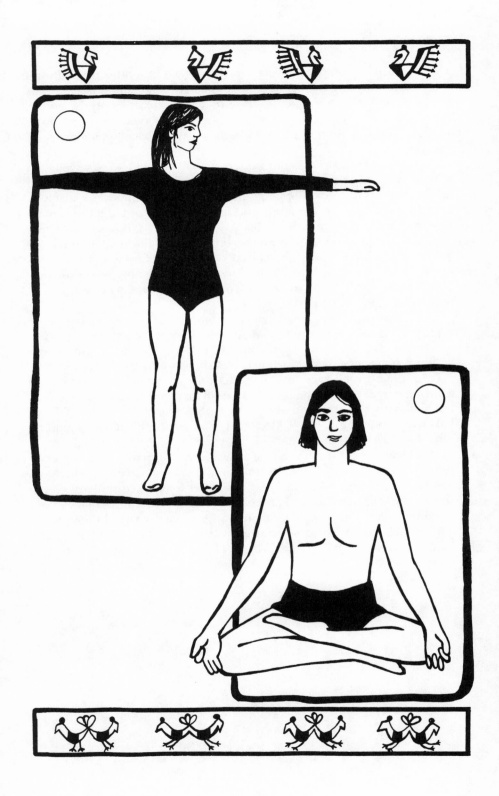

Chapter Five

Routine

Recipes make cooking easier. Healthful habits are part of the recipe for recreating yourself. When your Dhatus are in flux Ahamkara is less able to firmly identify with the body, and there are increased opportunities for illness to develop. Ayurveda believes that routine discipline for body and mind actively strengthens immunity by providing a foundation upon which Ahamkara can build a new you.

The Rishis who manifested Ayurveda determined long ago which habits were desirable and which should be avoided, and prepared daily and seasonal routines for people of varying prakrutis to follow for health maintenance. V people especially need routine because they are so innately irregular. V types find it very hard to stick to any routine for any length of time. K types love routine, but often their routines are unhealthy. They find as much difficulty in eliminating bad habits as Vs do in adding good ones. P types can add or remove habits almost at will, but they may have difficulty distinguishing between good and bad habits.

Many people are convinced that they have no time to allot to creating and following good habits. My teacher Vimalananda used to say, "Westerners wear their gods on their wrists." By this he meant that we allow an artificial, arrhythmic version of time to regulate our lives. All organisms require rhythm for proper functioning, but most of us ignore the natural internal and external rhythms which secretly influence us and try instead to create our own unnatural time. Our dedication to arbitrary schedules robs us of these rhythms, and weakens our ability to adapt to stresses. Fortunately, these rhythms can be regenerated by introducing additional routine into our lives. The human organism loves routine, and thrives when it is fed, exercised and rested regularly.

The need for discipline with regard to indulgence in food, sleep and sex is especially strong. Whatever your constitution, food, sleep and sex are the Three Pillars of your life, the three activities which when strong support the house which is your body. When they are weakened by misuse your house collapses. Since your health depends upon the support it receives from these Three Pillars, good food, sleep and sex habits are essential if you want to make a success of your life.

The Three Pillars represent digestion, rest, and creativity. Food is that which the body digests, which nourishes your organism. Overindulgence in food mainly aggravates Pitta, and leads to improper physical and mental digestion. Sleep is that which forces the mind to rest from its perpetual outward projection, and allows your personal identity to consolidate its control over your whole organism. Overindulgence in sleep mainly aggravates Kapha, and dulls the dynamism of body and mind. Sex is that which procreates, and allows you to temporarily merge with another being. Overindulgence in sex mainly aggravates Vata, and weakens your creativity and ability to communicate.

Properly consumed and digested food provides you the energy you require for creation, the projection of the uniqueness of your individuality into the environment. You may project your energy into matter to create an art form, or a balance sheet, or you may dissipate it by projecting it into unproductive activities like watching TV. If during the day you fail to either create with your energy or dissipate it, you will be tempted in the evening to project that energy into another human being during the sex act: to create another human form, to create satisfaction in your partner, or to simply dissipate it. After transmission you rest from your craving to project and express yourself and you enter the state of rest known as sleep, which prepares you for the next day's energy intake and expenditure. Digestion, creation, and rest are daily essentials for every healthy individual of any constitution. You need just enough food, sleep and sex; no more, and no less.

Most of us are too busy to follow all the suggestions listed in this chapter. Whatever you find useful for your own needs and aims, you should incorporate into your daily routine. A good routine improves health, which enhances your ability to perform your duties, accumulate possessions, and fulfill your desires.

Daily Routine

The morning routine helps prepare you to eat by purifying your organism of its wastes, the remains of that portion of the previous day's food which was rejected as unsatisfactory. All wastes must be eliminated before new fuel is added, just as ashes must be removed from a fireplace before a new fire is made. Wastes include urine, feces, sweat; all filth which accumulates on the sense organs; and all mental wastes like emotions, obsessions, and delusions. Salient points in this routine include:

ARISING

It is best to be awake for sunrise so that the body can begin to synchronize itself to the rhythm of the sun. Also, the last portion of the night is ruled by Vata, whose qualities of lightness and irregularity do not encourage good sound sleep. Since Vata is also involved in elimination, the pre-dawn period is the best time to try to eliminate the body's physical and mental wastes. Proper elimination also helps remove the Kapha that naturally accumulates overnight.

Vata's lightness also encourages good meditation. Sleep is a kind of death, a partial dissociation of the mind and spirit from the body. The sun's magnanimity in giving life by burning its own being to provide us with light and heat has induced many cultures to worship the sun as a deity. Everyone should rise early and marvel a few moments over the miracle of existence which is about to begin again, allowing this miracle to instill a deep-felt reverence for all life in the core of your being. Early morning is a good time to request Nature to maintain and amplify your own harmony during the day so that you will interact harmoniously with everyone and everything you encounter.

WASTES

Defecation once or twice daily is best. Three or more times a day unnecessarily increases Vata, the force which must expel the wastes, and encourages food to move through the gut too fast to be properly absorbed. Defecating immediately after a meal should not be encouraged, though it is wise to urinate immediately after each meal. Always clench your teeth tightly when voiding either urine or feces, to prevent Vata from loosening them.

Examine your urine and feces each morning and decide if they are healthy. Any disturbance in your wastes indicates poor digestion, and presence of Ama. To remedy this before it has an opportunity to sink deeply into your organism, do not eat anything, and drink only weak herbal tea, especially made of powdered ginger, until your wastes improve and your appetite intensifies. This is a general rule, and like all other generalities has its exceptions, but most of the time you should not put food into your system whenever your system shows signs of failing to digest it properly.

WASHING

Washing the hands, feet, face, mouth, eyes, and nose purifies the body's sense organs. You should first inspect your tongue. A coating on your tongue signifies a "coating" of poisonous Ama, undigested or improperly digested food material, in your digestive tract. A coating on the tongue may precede changes in the qualities of the wastes, so if you inspect your tongue regularly you may be able to prevent overt indigestion before it develops.

You should scrape your tongue daily, either with a tongue scraper or a spoon, using silver, copper or stainless steel. Scrape your tongue back to front slowly five to ten times to express as much filth from its crypts as possible. Occasional gargling of salt water with a pinch of turmeric added helps keep the gums, mouth and throat healthy.

Brush your teeth daily, but lightly, to prevent damage to tooth enamel or to gums. Indian toothbrushes were originally made of well-chewed twigs, which were used once and then thrown away. Modern research has proved that toothbrushes can harbor colonies of pathogenic bacteria, and that they may be one cause of recurrent infections. Keep your toothbrush clean and dry at all times, and replace it frequently.

Still used in rural India, twig toothbrushes floss your teeth as you brush. We Westerners must use dental floss. Daily flossing is important to dental health, as is daily use of tooth powder or toothpaste, whose primary purpose is to invigorate and purify the gums. A sample tooth powder recipe:

5 parts alum or alum root or white oak bark powder
3 parts black pepper powder
2 parts rock salt (the black salt known as Kala Namak or the white salt known as Sindhalu or Saindhav is best)
1 part turmeric powder
1/4 part natural camphor or clove oil

The eyes should be cleaned with warm water which has been held in the mouth a few moments to absorb some saliva. Saliva is good for the eyes. Once a week eye drops of honey, castor oil, rose water, or barberry or Triphala tea should be instilled to expel excess Kapha. The nose should be cleaned out with fresh water or lightly salted water and a drop of oil should be daily instilled into each nostril with the tip of the little finger. For both cleansing and lubrication (to forestall increase in Vata) two or three drops of oil should be instilled in each ear once every week or two.

MEDITATION

It is best to take a brief bath before meditating, but if this is inconvenient at least the hands, feet and face should be thoroughly washed. Meditating is a sort of eating, a consumption of subtle energies which are digested by the mind's subtle digestive fire. Meditation is a critical element of all daily programs because it satisfies the mind's hunger. Insufficient or improper meditation keeps the mind hungry, and makes it turn outward through its sense organs to seek satisfaction from sense objects, including especially physical food.

Use of food to satisfy the mind alone without consideration for the body always leads to disease. Good meditation nourishes the organism so thoroughly that the body can maintain itself on less food. Control of desire, which is mental hunger, is the key to longevity and immortality.

Anything can be a meditation, as long as it is sincere and heartfelt. From the strict viewpoint of the health of the organism, the simplest of all meditations involves the sun, without whose heat and light we could not exist. Of all hues, the golden color of the sun is healthiest, most nourishing and most productive of strength and vigor. Ayurveda advises daily ingestion of the gold color.

Yogis often gather this golden color by staring at the sun just as it comes over the horizon each day for a few minutes, meditating on the solar magnificence and munificence. Anyone can do this safely; once the sun's brightness reaches a point of uncomfortable intensity, you close your eyes and continue to stare for a few more moments through your closed eyelids. Even a few minutes a day will invigorate your being, and improve your vision.

If you are wary of the sun, or live in a cloudy climate, you can obtain gold by the Ayurvedic method of staring into a golden bowl filled with cow's ghee (clarified butter), which is golden in color. Or you can use the procedure called Trataka, in which you place at arm's length at eye level a lamp containing ghee, which burns with a golden light, and stare fixedly into it until tears come. Or, you can close your eyes and visualize the sun, or a glowing ball of hot gold. After any of these procedures the eyes should be washed and a drop or two of pure rose water instilled into each one to remove any excess heat.

MASSAGE

Touch is the skin's sense. The skin and the digestive tract are the physical barriers which separate you from your environment. They control entrance into your system, permitting nutrients inside while refusing entry to pathogens. Bodily wastes can also be excreted through both the skin and the gut. When excretion through other channels becomes inefficient the excess is directed out through the skin. Skin disease usually develops when the skin is clogged with toxic wastes. The health of the skin is thus intimately connected with the health of the digestive tract. Skin disease improves when digestive function improves, and when the skin is cleansed of all its impurities and toned to vibrancy the digestive tract also becomes healthier.

Every human being needs regular oil massage. While self-massage is adequate for most people most of the time, everyone should seek professional massage from time to time. Massage makes the skin soft and unctuous and controls Vata by reducing Vata's cold, dry, light, rough and erratic qualities. Its rhythmic motion allays joint and muscle stiffness and makes all body movements free and rhythmic. The circulation of the blood increases, encouraging quicker removal of metabolic wastes. Massage also relaxes the body prior to more vigorous exercise.

V people require massage more than do P and K types because the sense of touch is most acute in V people, so acute that touch can sometimes be painful. Touch can also be therapeutic. V people need to be touched more than do others because touch helps ground them in a level of consciousness appropriate for living in the world. Massage provides therapeutic touch, and softens the acuteness of the sense of touch.

V people are also more prone to damage by radiation than are other types, and research has shown that vegetable oil in the diet and applied to the skin helps protect individuals from the destructive effects of radiation. The internal and external use of medicated oils is the fundamental method used by Ayurveda to balance V people and manage Vata-caused conditions.

To protect their health and sanity all V people should visit a competent masseur or masseuse regularly, not less than once a month, if possible on the same day of the week each time at the same time of day. Routine reinforces and enhances the massage's effects.

P individuals should go for variety in massage, sampling shiatsu, accupressure, polarity, and various other techniques to keep their minds occupied. P tissues are inherently tender and irritable and should be manipulated with care to avoid aggravation.

K types require firm hands, deeply penetrating fingers, and a technique bordering on harshness to awaken the sluggish circulation and eliminate cellular wastes. They should use oil sparingly or dispense with it altogether. People of dual constitutions should select massage based on the season of the year and their own individual conditions.

It is best to use oil from a plant which grows or could grow in your area. You should select the oil according to season (heating oils like mustard or sesame in the winter and cooling oils like coconut or olive in the summer), climate (wet oils like sesame and castor in dry climates and drying oils like safflower in a wet climate), and individual constitution. Sandalwood oil is probably the best of all medicinal oils because it reduces the Pitta and Kapha-causing properties of any oils it may be mixed with, and because it promotes mental balance and coolness.

All oils are good for V people, but sesame, almond, mustard and castor are usually best. Olive oil, cocoa butter and coconut oil are optimal for Ps, with some fragrant oil like lavender or sandalwood added. Ks should avoid oil and concentrate on dry massage, but for skin lubrication they can apply sunflower, safflower or, in winter, mustard oils. VP people need less oil than do pure Vs, but can use most oils and should get regular massages. PKs should usually use sunflower or corn oil, and VKs can use mustard, almond, sunflower or corn as they please, and should get frequent massages.

For general body massage an ounce of an aromatic oil like sandalwood can be mixed with a quart of an oil appropriate for current conditions. V, VP and VK types with poor circulation to the extremities may choose to add one to two teaspoons of oil of wintergreen or eucalyptus oil per quart of their main oil. Pine needle oil helps combat tendencies to muscle spasm, and pure jasmine oil, as much as one ounce per pint, can be used for an aphrodisiac effect. Unmedicated vegetable oils except castor oil should never be applied to rheumatic joints. Castor oil can be applied to any part of the skin at any time. A little oil of garlic in the castor oil to act as a counter-irritant helps the rheumatic part cleanse itself.

Never use mineral oil or oil perfumed or colored with chemicals on your body; the skin eats oil as surely as if you had put it into your mouth. Store your natural, cold-pressed oil for body massage in the refrigerator, but do not preserve it longer than three months. If you store your oil in a red bottle and expose it to the sun daily for forty days its heat increases which makes it more efficient for use in Vata and Vata-Kapha diseases like body aches and pains. Storing oil in a blue bottle and exposing it to the sun daily for forty days makes it cooler, which enhances its effects on prickly heat, burns, and other high-heat Pitta conditions.

Follow the flow of body energy when you massage yourself to avoid diverting Vata from its normal direction. You can do this by working in the direction that the hairs grow. Work from the hands and feet towards the trunk, and from outwards inward. Apply a little extra oil over the body's vital parts—the heart, navel, genitals, joints, anus, and any as yet unoiled sense organs—and apply it liberally over all hairy areas, like your head, armpits, pubes, and chest. The hair's nutrition is linked with the nutrition of the bones. Oil on your head hair also helps control Vata in your mind. Once a week work some oil into your scalp and wait twenty minutes or so for it to soak in before you wash it out. Oil massage of the head relaxes both brain and body and strengthens the sense organs.

When you have no time to massage your whole body at least massage the soles of your feet. Oil massage of the feet promotes sound sleep. If your eyes are weak, oil both your great toenails nightly. Avoid massage when your digestive tract is full of Ama. Abnormal bodily wastes and a heavily coated tongue indicate Ama even if there are no other symptoms, but most acute diseases, especially fevers, are associated with extensive Ama.

EXERCISE

Exercise may be passive like massage, active like aerobics, or both passive and active like Yoga postures. Exercise increases the body's stamina and resistance to disease, by facilitating the action of the immune system. It clears all channels, promotes circulation and waste disposal, and destroys fat. Regular exercise even reduces anxiety and produces a sense of well-being by stimulating the release of endorphins, which explains why exercise can be addictive.

V people become addicted to vigorous exercise because it temporarily exhausts them, preventing them from thinking at their normal hyper-speed rate, and because the endorphins increase the organism's pain threshold, which is important to the normally pain-sensitive V person. Excessive vigorous exercise exhausts the body, which disturbs Vata.

Also, the dullness of mind which vigorous exercise engenders is only temporary. The rebound effect makes the mind work even more vigorously and chaotically afterwards, as if to make up for lost time.

V people are often most attracted to running or jogging, which puts great pressure on their inherently weak joints. Joint injuries in V people are more likely to become complicated or to result in arthritis than similar injuries in other types. Some Vs are attracted to sports like handball which require intense bursts of energy, which Vs have in abundance; the ultimate result, however, is total energy wipeout. Mild, regular exercise, such as Yoga, Tai Chi, walking, or swimming, is always better for V people than intense exertion. Yoga and Tai Chi are especially good for V types because being contemplative they promote mental equanimity.

Vs tend to be fidgety anyway, and the energy a confirmed fidgeter burns off in a day is equivalent to that expended in jogging several miles. Rhythmic exercise is always better for V types than are chaotic workouts. For example, regular weight training with light weights is far better for V types than sporadic aerobic exhaustion. Rebounders are good for V people who are addicted to jogging and running. Participatory exercise like folk dancing may also satisfy these requirements.

Since V people hate routines and love to try new things, they may begin with any sort of exercise they please. Once they have created an exercise habit they should then tone down the vigor and enhance the stabilization. External sources of heat like steam baths and hot tubs further stimulate the circulation. VP people require less heat than do pure Vs but should generally observe V-type exercise guidelines.

P people love vigorous exercise like weightlifting because it feeds their aggressiveness and makes them all the more intense, irritable and driven. Competitive sports like tennis excite them because they are naturally competitive and love the thrill of competition. An optimal exercise for a P person provides this competitiveness without permitting it to reinforce the natural P egotism. Team sports like basketball and volleyball, in which cooperation is emphasized and individual heroics are downplayed, or sports like backpacking which permit you to compete against yourself, are best for P types. Tai Chi and Yoga can be good for Ps if they use them to cool their fire and balance their aggression.

Ps should indulge in external sources of heat with care. If Nature had meant Ps to lie for hours in the sun, She would have given them dark skins. Ps should use a sun blocking lotion with this in mind, and should go under cover when they begin to get too warm. Swimming is great for Ps because it is cooling; it helps reduce fire, as do water skiing and snow skiing. Swimming is an excellent, simple form of exercise which is especially good for Vs and Ps but is suitable for everyone.

K people really *need* vigorous exercise. Many K people need strenuous encouragement to develop an exercise habit, but once it develops the K person will normally stick with it. Ks usually do not like to have to involve themselves intensively with the activity, and so tend to choose exercises like bicycling which can be done on autopilot. Such repetitive activities reinforce the repetitive, habitual nature of the K organism, however. Strenuous sports, or complicated aerobic routines, are better. Yoga and Tai Chi can be good if they are used to stimulate and energize the organism.

K and PK types alone should indulge in activities which strain the physical organism to its limits, like ice hockey or lumberjacking. Most VKs do not have the same inherent stamina because of the influence of Vata. They require vigorous exercise regularly but not continuously, and need liberal doses of heat. Though Ks should avoid repetitive exercise, as in the case of V people K types who need to be motivated to exercise can begin with repetitive activities like long-distance running or calisthenics, and complexity can gradually be added to the program.

Exercise cannot benefit you if you work yourself to the point of exhaustion. Ayurveda's rule is that you should never exert more than half your capacity. If you know you will be exhausted after, say, one hour of bicycling, you should never cycle more than half an hour at a time. In extreme climates, when your energy is dissipated faster, it should be even less than half-capacity. Do not exercise when you are ill with respiratory diseases, such as chronic cough or cold, or when you have any severe inflammation or severe indigestion. Children should not begin strenuous exercise too early in life, nor should strenuous exercise be continued into old age.

Wrongful exercise can put body parts out of balance with one another, overemphasizing one area while neglecting others. Even appropriate exercise can have undesirable effects when overdone. Vigorous exercise increases the need for physical food to replace the nutrients burned to supply energy. This extra food requires extra energy for digestion. Since this energy must be obtained at the mind's expense, over-exercising dulls the mind. Ayurveda always encourages meditative exercise, like Yoga and Tai Chi, to prevent this mental dullness and to ensure proper energy flow throughout the organism. Such practices regularize V people, calm P people, invigorate K people, and help integrate those with dual constitutions.

Ayurveda suggests that exercise be performed with rhythmic breathing. Breathing brings the life force (known as Prana in Sanskrit) into the body, and removes gaseous wastes from it. Good breathing purifies the lungs; poor breathing makes the lungs unhealthy, and disturbs the colon and the bones. To make your exercise effective your breath must flow regularly, evenly and deeply.

The simplest breathing exercise you can do is to sit and concentrate on breathing from deep in your abdomen, slowing the flow gradually and effortlessly until you are taking only a few breaths each minute.

The Sun Salute - Surya Namaskara

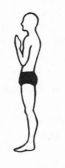

With your palms together, stand quietly and inhale and exhale slowly.

Brings your palms apart as you inhale slowly stretching your arms and head back. With your arms open and the palms facing upwards, arch back easily.

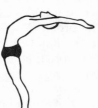

Exhale slowly keeping your head between your arms and bend forward from the waist slowly. Keeping your knees straight as you go down relax the head, neck, shoulders and arms, and touch the floor with your hands if possible.

Bending both knees, place your palms flat on either side of your feet. Stretch the right leg back keeping your right knee and toe on the floor. Inhale slowly as you stretch your chin upwards.

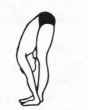

Bring your feet parallel to each other and raise your hips up into a jack-knife position forming a triangle with your chin locked to your chest. Retain the breath.

Move your feet back and lower yourself until your toes, knees, chest, and forehead, but not your abdomen, are touching the floor. Exhale slowly as you lower yourself.

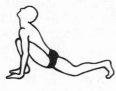

Inhale slowly as you easily arch back the spine with your chin up, hips and toes on the floor and the elbows slightly bent.

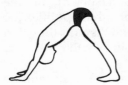

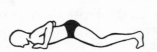

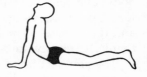

Exhale slowly as you raise your hips into a jack-knife position forming a triangle. Keep your heels to the floor with the chin locked to the chest.

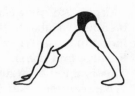

Inhale slowly as your bring your left leg up between both hands. Keep your right knee on the floor and your palms flat with your chin up.

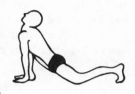

Exhale slowly as you bring both feet together, knees straight, bending forward from the hips. Relax your neck, head, and arms.

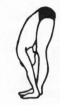

Slowly raise up inhaling as you stretch your hands outwards then upwards arching back your arms and head with the palms upward.

Exhale slowly while bringing your palms together and closing your eyes.

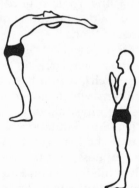

Carefully observe the different changes in your body: the increase of heat, your breath, your heart beat.

Each of the twelve postures should be held three seconds at first. Once you become familiar with the Sun Salute each asana (posture) will flow one into the other. There should be no feeling of breathlessness, but above all, go slowly according to your own to your own capacity. If you have a history of high blood pressure or heart trouble, please check with your physician before you do this exercise.

Yogis say that each individual is born with a specified number of breaths available to them, and as soon as these breaths are used up the individual dies. The faster you breathe, the sooner you use up your breaths, and the shorter your life. You live longer by breathing slower. This is another argument against excessive vigorous aerobic exercise. Whatever your exercise or meditation, you should concentrate on your breathing for a few minutes each day, sitting with your back straight and breathing with your abdomen, not your chest.

My teacher Vimalananda used to say that even if you ignore all other rules of routine you can still maintain good health as long as you:

Keep your bowels moving (keep your colon clean)
Keep your body moving (exercise regularly)
Keep your breath moving (always breathe slowly and deeply).

Even if you never do stringent Ayurvedic or Yogic purifications, you should take the time every day to make sure that your colon empties itself properly. Even if you only take the time to walk around the block, do push-ups on the living room floor, or do isometric exercises in the bedroom, you should take out five to ten minutes each day, preferably at the same time daily, to move your body. Even if you never study Pranayama, the Yogic science of breathing, you should spend at least five minutes a day breathing quietly, deeply, and slowly, to regenerate your stores of Prana.

The crest jewel of exercises is the Sun Salutation, or Surya Namaskara, a sequence of Yogic postures performed with rhythmic breathing. Each posture has associated with it a Mantra, a specialized sound pattern which invigorates the subtle body as the posture invigorates the physical body. The breathing helps tie the two bodies together. The Sun Salutation is balancing and harmonizing even if you do not know the Mantras, however, because it helps to integrate all the various identities (spiritual, mental, and physical) into one. It is simultaneously a meditation and an exercise.

The Sun Salutation is deceptively simple in appearance. You should begin with one to three rounds daily, and work up to a dozen or more, according to how long it takes you to do each one. It should be performed slowly and meditatively by V people, quickly and vigorously by K people, and at a medium pace by P people. P people especially should learn the appropriate Mantras for each movement, to help engage their active intelligences. Allow your breath to flow freely as your body shifts from pose to pose.

The Sun Salutation is the supreme exercise because it balances and activates the body, controls and conditions the mind, and possesses a spiritual aspect as well. It is a salute to the sun, the source of our life. Even if you cannot work the Sun Salutation into your daily routine, no V is so disorganized, no P is so busy, and no K is so indolent that they cannot do some kind of exercise. You can at the least always walk, an exercise which tones the bowels, relaxes the body, and promotes digestion, all the while preserving mental clarity. If all else fails you can laugh. Laughter burns calories, improves lung function, oxygenates the blood, invites Prana into the system, releases endorphins, and strengthens the immune system. And it is so easy to do!

BATHING

Ayurveda advocates the warm water bath; Yoga advises the use of cold water. The body cools minutes after exposure to hot water as the blood vessels which dilated with heat contract in reaction. A cold shower has the opposite effect, making you warm within a few minutes as the vessels constricted by the cold dilate.

A good compromise for V people, who require heat, is to luxuriate in a warm bath or shower, and after imbibing enough heat to feel warm, to rinse at the end with cold water to help them preserve the warmth. P people should if possible adapt themselves to cool showers and baths, to help remove their excess heat. K types should adapt to cool water, to invigorate themselves. No one should bathe for at least an hour after eating to avoid drawing blood away from the gut where it is required for digestion. Bathing should be temporarily avoided in case of diarrhea, distention, chronic cold, indigestion, and in most acute diseases in which Ama predominates.

Intensely hot water applied directly to the head drains strength from the sense organs. While shampoo may be used regularly for the hair and scalp, soap should be used on the body only in case of real grime, as it robs the skin of its protective mantle and encourages the growth of bacteria which cause body odor. Soap is especially bad for mucus membranes (anus, genitals, nipples, etc.). Instead of soap, clay or barley or chickpea flour should be used to soak up the oil left after the massage and the sweat left after the exercise. Also, flour draws out the wastes excreted by the system after massage and exercise and tones the skin without drying it or leaving a soap film. Soap should never be used on most skin diseases.

If you have not applied oil to your whole body you can incorporate oil into the paste. Mix half a cup of oil with a cup of chickpea, barley or even wheat flour, and add one-quarter to one-half teaspoon of turmeric powder to assist in skin purification. Add just enough water to make it a thick but spreadable paste and apply it evenly, rubbing it in as you apply. If possible let it dry until it begins to crack. This acts as a mask, or pack, for the whole body.

A mental bath should always accompany the physical bath, to awaken the mind and enkindle its digestive fires. In India specific Mantras have been allocated for this purpose. Devotional songs, hymns, or in fact any song or chant which you enjoy will help satisfy your mind, and will make for a more satisfying bath.

Lifestyle

It is good to perform your routine in the morning before you go out into the world, because it applies "armor" to you for your foray into the external environment. Failure to properly shield yourself against the dangers of the outside world opens you to invasion by destabilizing outside forces, be they humans or bacteria, since every interaction with another being affects your personality. This "armor" does not insulate you from beneficial energies; it merely allows you to screen incoming influences to decide which you would like to take. By selecting beneficial experiences and shielding yourself against divisive forces you can create for yourself an environment which will be conducive to your total health, according to your own personal constitution.

CLOTHING

Your clothes are the removable part of your external armor. Today clothes are more important than ever, given the preponderance of evil influences circulating in society. Your clothing should always be light and airy, made of natural fibers like cotton, wool or linen. Silk is the fabric which best insulates against adverse external influences too subtle to be otherwise avoided. This is why Indian priests like to use silk clothing during ritual worship. Some authorities say that rayon also possesses this property.

Always wear clean clothes, and never wear clothing, flowers or footwear which anyone else has worn, since these items too easily pick up an individual's innate personality vibrations. No one's vibration is better for you than your own, except that of a saint, someone who has reached a higher level of integration than you. Use of a saint's clothing, flowers, or footwear actually helps harmonize your being.

In India people lovingly worship both the feet and the footwear of their saints, because they know that energy is brought into the body through the crown of the head and exits through the soles of the feet by extracting abnormal heat from the system. Applying henna leaf paste or rubbing ghee with a small bronze bowl on the soles of the feet can reduce fever. The energy which exits from you will be polluted and miasmic if you are unhealthy mentally or physically, or it will be tonic and healthful if you are well-balanced and integrated, as saints are. Your footwear absorbs much of this energy.

Footwear is not allowed in the house in India or other Oriental countries because no matter how clean it is externally it still traps some of this polluted energy and pollutes whatever it comes in contact with, just as muddy shoes track up a clean floor. Since your own use of your own footwear affects your consciousness adversely to some extent, it is best to go barefoot whenever possible, especially inside the house. Another reason to go barefoot is that shoe leather itself, being the skin of a dead animal, pollutes the consciousness. Shoes made out of rubber are an improvement but they adversely affect the eyes. Strict Indian Yogis always wear wooden sandals.

EMPLOYMENT

Work consumes at least a third of our lives. Success or failure at your chosen profession affects your self-confidence, your self-worth, and the self-validity of your personality. Your work should agree with your prakruti.

V people love to work at jobs which require sudden bursts of intense energy, because they naturally work that way. Such work exhausts them, however, and should be avoided. Even though they despise and resist anything boring, repetitive or routine, ideal employment for a V is somewhat repetitive, to discipline the normally erratic V nature. V people should avoid places where the air is exceptionally cool and dry, such as the clean room of an electronics manufacturing outfit, or exceptionally dusty, like a feed or fertilizer mill, even though such work would be routine.

Vs need a soothing home and work environment to smooth out their rough edges. They need adequate rest, and should arrange for a 10-minute afternoon catnap if possible because afternoon is the Vata time of day. Vs should not schedule important meetings for late afternoon unless they want to sleep through them. V people must pace themselves carefully and resist the temptation to try to do everything at once. It is sometimes acutely painful for V people to be steady or endure tedium, but it is essential for them to do so.

V types are excellent original thinkers, and if they theorize for a living they must be sure to keep themselves grounded with a fixed routine of massage, exercise, sleep, and food. This also applies to those Vs who because of their love of frequent change are led into travel-related professions, like the airlines. Any V person who wishes to enjoy the constant stimulation of such a job, the continual excitement of seeing new places and meeting new people, must observe strict control over all other aspects of his or her life. Change and excitement are intoxicants for V people, and like all other intoxicants they are meant for occasional indulgence only. The challenge is to find a job which has sufficient excitement to hold a Vs interest but is sufficiently routine to prevent imbalances.

P people are practical to a fault. They take ideas dreamed up by V theoreticians and apply them to real situations. Ps are realists and enjoy the palpabilities of reality; for example, they tend to be obsessed with numbers and with time, like how many new accounts can be obtained per month, or how many appointments can be squeezed into one eight-hour day. Ps are by nature aggressive and self-promoting. To them everything is a contest, and all contests are meant to be won. They must be in the forefront of all activity, first across the finish line in any competition. They invite as many stimuli into their lives as they can cram in, and demand perfect functioning from their bodies at all times.

Ideal employment for Ps would include sufficient challenge to keep them occupied without the stress of severe competition. Teaching, for example, provides a P with the intellectual challenge of communicating his or her knowledge to others, but need not lead to perpetual comparison with others in the same profession, as a career in sales might. Ps ought also to avoid physically irritating work situations, like welding or metal casting which involve intense heat that might increase Pitta. Violence of any kind is not good for Ps, even in the movies.

P people who do choose stimulating employment always struggle against irritability and impatience. Ps love to plan and become enthusiastic about their plans; they do not take obstacles or delays well. They need to be willing to listen to other people and to refrain from dismissing their ideas out of hand. At mid-day, the Pitta time of day, Ps become exceptionally hungry and irritable and should avoid confrontations before they are able to eat. Ps find it hard to separate their professions from their private lives. No one should take their work home with them, but P people must be stricter than others in this separation of career and family. They need to set aside time to "waste," to make themselves available to their families for seemingly non-essential pursuits.

Ks are not known as either original thinkers or outstanding engineers, but a good K makes a great administrator. The innate K stability and balance makes any business they are associated run as if on "greased wheels." A K whose position is almost totally routine and repetitive must consciously inject change and stimulation into his or her life. Even if it was only a rearrangement of furniture in the office or the home, any effort to frequently change their physical environment is therapeutic for K types, who should also ensure that if their work is not physically active their leisure time is. Competition is good for them, although they may find it stressful, and they should avoid accepting neat, tidy answers to complex problems, even in unimportant matters.

Morning is the Kapha time of day, and Ks should not expect to be able to do much creative work then. They should keep the mornings for routine work, which Ks can do better than anyone else, and tackle thornier questions around mid-day or in the afternoon when the cosmos provides them Pitta for decision-making power and Vata to encourage speculation, respectively. Making your constitution work for you, not against you, in every aspect of your life is one of life's great challenges.

PETS

Pets are extensions of their owners' personalities, small versions of their masters. Most people prefer pets with whom they can innately relate, who reflect their own character traits, but it is better to keep a pet who is therapeutic for your own imbalances. V people do well with dogs, for example, because a canine's lovable, sloppy, openheartedness warms, reassures, relaxes and stabilizes the Vs cold, fearful, fickle nature. K individuals do better with small animals like birds because an avian's light, bright cheerfulness helps offset some of a Ks natural ponderousness, sluggishness and fixity.

Some K people find large dogs beneficial because both dog and owner need vigorous exercise, and responsibility for the canine encourages the K person to exercise along with the dog. Some V types do well with small furry high-strung animals like guinea pigs and hamsters which elicit maternal instinct from their owners.

P personalities are sometimes too overbearing to obtain much incentive for self-development from the simpler personalities of birds and beasts. Ps should not take the easy way out and select an animal who is too easy to get along with, nor one who is so aggressive that the two beings feed off one another's instincts to violence. A large long-lived bird like a parrot may be complex enough to demand attention from a P, but cats, who have strongly-held opinions about most subjects including their masters, present continuous challenges to the probing P mind and make perhaps the best P pets. The P has to keep up with the feline, and this is a refreshingly new experience for many hotshot Ps.

SPOUSE

Just as you would not throw out a pet who did not perfectly meet your needs, you should not throw out a spouse who is not a perfect match for you. But you will be benefitted if you know something of your constitution before you select either a pet or a spouse.

Ancient Indian sexology insists that individuals of like constitution be paired together—Vs with Vs, Ps with Ps, and Ks with Ks—because of their inherent sexual proclivities. For example, Ks are not particularly oversexed but do become quite lusty once their natural indolence is conquered. Because of their innate physical strength two Ks will not easily wear each other out with their persistent readiness for intercourse. Two V partners excite each other easily and become easily exhausted, which is fine, since there is a sense of mutuality present. A V and a K paired together might experience mutual frustration: first the V would feel lack of interest from the partner, then after days or weeks when the Ks sexual appetite was awakened and became ravenous the V would be too worn out to respond with equal ardor.

Ayurvedic wisdom adds that like types make better mates because of similar mental processes and attitudes. V people cannot hold onto money, for example; they fritter it away, or donate it to some "cause." P people calculate well, plan, and save and spend with conscious design. A pure P and a pure V married to one another would probably tear out their mutual hair over the partner's fiscal habits.

Unfortunately, two people of like dispositions are likely to have like defects. Two V people living together will tend to feed off one another's chaotic energies and will often end up bouncing off the walls, babbling at one another in blue streaks without much communication. Two K people could conceivably so immobilize each other that they could live together for years with little interaction. Two P people will rarely be able to resist competing against one another, trying to gain the upper hand in the relationship. Their habitual mutual irritation can lead to great and terrible tussles interspersed with periods of uneasy truce.

Prakruti is the problem. Recall that Kapha is the force which forces Water and Earth to cooperate together, even though they would prefer to ignore one another. At the core of their beings K people feel a desire to avoid confrontation and no effort from within or without can completely overcome that tendency. Even if a lone K can exert sufficient will force to encourage self-transformation, it is too easy for two Ks living together to persist in their old habits and reinforce each other's innate tendencies.

Likewise, heat is not the only reason for a Ps inborn antagonism. Pitta's job is to balance two mutually antagonistic elements: Fire and Water. Two P people living together are almost certain to project antagonism at one another; it comes naturally. Two Vs in the same household are unlikely ever to develop the discipline they so urgently need, because Vata has to try to impose limitation on Air, which resists all limitation, with the help of Ether, which can exert only an ethereal influence. Two people of like prakruti always tend to reinforce one another's constitutional weaknesses.

Ps can give Vs organization for their mental chaos, and Vs can give Ps continuous communication challenges. But if there is imbalance, the V wind will blow like a bellows on the P fire and incinerate the relationship, or the P fire will heat up the V air and expand it like a balloon until it flies off or bursts. Vs can get stability and balance from Ks, and shake them out of their ponderousness in return, or because of their mutual coldness the V air will solidify K into stubbornness, or the K stickiness will obstruct Vs free flow. Ps heat up and activate Ks; Ks cool and ballast Ps. If the P is too hot, though, the K will boil over, and if the K is too wet the P will get drowned.

Two people who live together long enough begin to rub off on one another, and even begin to look like one another. Any two people who sleep next to one another nightly enter each other's aura, even if there is no sexual relationship between them, because of the proximity and the lowering of defenses which occurs during sleep. Proximity may in some cases be enough to promote integration, if the couple involved is committed to the relationship, but the force of Nature is often too strong to overcome with good intentions alone. For example, because Fire is lacking in their relationship, a V-K match is unlikely to succeed without a significant area of shared interest, like a job or a hobby, to provide the personality welding which is needed to make a marriage a success.

The whole issue becomes much murkier when VP, PK and VK permutations are added. A VP mated with a PK forms one of the most stable of relationships, because both have enough Fire energy to communicate with one another, and the V of the one balances the K of the other. A VK and a PK can form a good match, though their shared K stubbornness will tend to amplify the differences between them. A VK and a VP may make a good spiritual pair, but the stability of their mundane life will be reduced because of the shared V influence.

Your choice must fundamentally depend on your ambitions for relationship in this lifetime. If you want a stable relationship with a compatible spouse, select someone of your own constitutional type. The mutual excess which occurs in such pairings is easier to endure than the strained dynamic inherent in a pairing of two people whose constitutions differ radically. Two constitutionally similar individuals involved with one another intuitively understand the forces which motivate their partners, because those same forces motivate them. If you do not want to have to put a lot of energy into a relationship, look for a spouse who is of your metabolic type.

If you wish to use a relationship as a vehicle for self-evolution, select a partner who will stimulate you and shake you up, who will offer you what you lack and to whom you can provide complementary energy. Be warned, though, that such a course may find you and your spouse eating, drinking, and being merry in widely differing ways as a result of the constitutional variance.

SURROUNDINGS

The above rules hold for all interpersonal interactions. Also, the friends and comrades you select for yourself should be selected with the harmonizing effect of their influence as chief criterion. Friendship with self-destructive individuals will magnify any self-destructiveness you have not yet expunged from your being; camaraderie with the empathetic will increase your own empathy. When you choose to associate yourself with any individual, you should be aware of the effects that person has on your own personality. Association with negative individuals, or Sanga Dosha, causes you to pick up physical, mental and spiritual defects from them while Satsanga, association with strong, healthy, spiritual people allows their harmoniousness to rub off on you.

Physical and mental characteristics should also influence your choice of residence. Pure V people do best in hot, humid climates like Hawaii and the Gulf Coast, and find cold climates almost unbearable. Pure K people require hot, arid climates like the Western desert to balance themselves, and pure P types shun torrid climates and adore the cold. V and K people both need regular exposure to the sun, though overexposure can damage the immune system. Ps must be wary of the sun.

Socially and culturally, you might choose to make your home in as opulent a neighborhood as possible, with neighbors of like minds and like tastes, and avoid any contact with poverty to prevent your sensibilities from being disturbed by unsettling sights. This attitude would maximize your ability to manifest your own physical wealth and would enhance your Earth and Water energies.

You might, if you chose to maximize your spiritual nature, live in a simple and limited style in a simple dwelling with simple friends as neighbors, avoiding the company of the rich and powerful whose minds are immersed in the mire of the world. This would enhance the Air and Ether energies in your organism.

And if you want to exercise your mental faculties, you could adapt yourself to whatever environment you found yourself in, experiencing people of all sorts and styles, maintaining under all circumstances perfect presence of mind. This would strengthen your Fire energy.

Varied vegetables cook together into a stew, each offering part of its own individuality and each accepting part of the identity of the others. Just as you have a responsibility to yourself to eat healthily and to live healthily, you have the responsibility of choosing healthy associates, healthy environments, and healthy pastimes. This is why Ayurveda insists that all your spare time should be spent with your "elders." An elder is anyone who is older than you in maturity and experience; chronological age is irrelevant. The society which has no elders must be shunned, no matter how advanced materially or artistically it may be.

SLEEP

Sleep is known in Ayurveda as the "Wet-nurse of the World" because it nourishes beings with motherliness and promotes proper growth. Sleep is bodily inertia with mental relaxation; it is closely associated with Kapha because its essence is inertia.

Night is the time for sleep, after the personality tires of projecting itself externally. Ten-minute catnaps are good for V types. Long naps are permitted in the peak of summer, when days are hot and nights are short. Otherwise sleeping during the day increases Kapha, and only the very young, the very old, the very weak and those exhausted by sex, intoxicants, disease, travel, overwork or other physical or emotional trauma should nap longer than ten or fifteen minutes in an afternoon. Sometimes a nap before eating will benefit a case of acute indigestion, but usually, unless you have been awake all night, sleeping during the day inevitably produces Ama.

Evening is the Kapha time of night, when Ks must struggle against becoming cozily inert. Midnight is the Pitta time of night. Ps especially should not be awake then, since their appetites will grow and they will be tempted to eat. Ps sometimes wake up in the middle of the night hungry or, if they have ulcers, in pain from the acid Pitta has caused the body to secrete then. The hours just before dawn are governed by Vata, another reason why V people should go to bed early, when Kapha will encourage them to sleep soundly, and arise in the early morning, when Vata will not permit them sound sleep anyway.

No one should consume a full physical or mental meal less than two hours before bed, except supplements when necessary to promote sleep. All physical and mental digestive processes should be complete before surrendering to sleep. Meditation, or nervine herbs like valerian, may help you get to sleep. V people often find a cup of warm milk with a pinch of saffron in it to be soporific.

Sitting up is the best sleeping position, because it provides the most alert sleep. Sleeping on the right side is the most relaxing; on the left, most digestive; on your back, disturbing to Vata; and on your stomach, disturbing of everything. Yogis who do not sleep sitting up prefer to sleep on the right side because this encourages the function of the left nostril by suppressing breathing through the right nostril. This cools and relaxes the body making it easier to control, which is essential for Yoga.

Individuals who wish to amply enjoy the pleasures of the world should sleep on their left sides, since this promotes functioning of the right nostril by obstructing free flow through the left. The right nostril heats and activates the body, and increases the organism's interest in food, sleep and sex. This assists you to better externalize your personality to enable it to better enjoy sensuousness.

Sleeping on the back allows both nostrils to function together, which discourages body-mind-spirit integration and indirectly promotes disease by encouraging energy to leave the body. Sleeping on the stomach promotes disease directly by obstructing deep, healthy breathing.

It is best to sleep with the crown of your head into the east and your feet into the west; this promotes meditative sleep. Sleeping with your head into the north draws energy out of the body, disturbing body-mind-spirit integration. If your head is into the south energy is drawn into your body, improving your health. Your head into the west promotes disturbing dreams. Recent research in India supports the relaxing effects of east and the disturbing effects of north.

You should always wash your hands, feet and face, massage your feet with a little oil, and meditate for a few moments to allow the day's negativity to dissipate before entering into the arms of sleep. If you have trouble with frequent wet dreams, washing your legs and feet in cold water before retiring will draw energy away from the genitals and reduce the likelihood of a nocturnal emission.

You should go to bed only to sleep, never to read, write or think, and you should arise immediately on waking. Never sleep in a kitchen or any other place where food is prepared, since both the savory odors and the subtle vibrations in the area will alert your digestive tract and disturb your sleep.

The ideal form of sleep is called Yoga Nidra, a state of complete physical inertness with retention of mental alertness and awareness. The more perfectly you can approach this ideal, the better prepared your organism will be for its new incarnation at dawn, when your routine begins again.

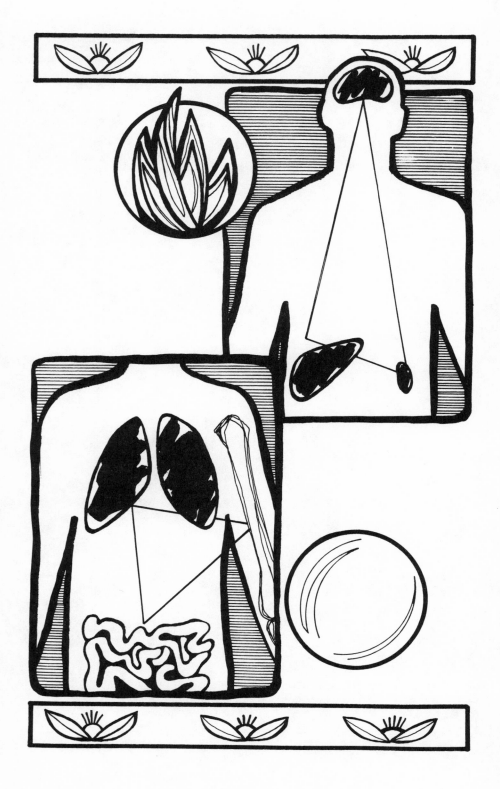

Chapter Six
Balance

Structure in life helps reduce the effects of stress on the organism. Stress, or rather improper reaction to stress, can cause diseases such as angina pectoris and asthma, and can worsen pre-existent disease. Scientific studies have shown that stress can increase blood cholesterol and stomach acid, and can aggravate cancer, viral infections, and rheumatoid arthritis. Stress is known to impair the immune system's ability to respond to invasion, thus permitting alien beings like viruses and cancerous cells to proliferate. When the nervous system is stimulated by the emotions which result from the stress it may even encourage the alien cells to spread.

Stress occurs every time you have to adapt to a new situation. Every time your environment—your physical, mental, emotional, social and spiritual surroundings—changes, you must change along with it and develop a new equilibrium with it. Your resilience, which is your capacity to roll with the punches and snap back to normal after even the lowest of blows, is your immunity. As stress increases, strain on your immune system grows. When the strain becomes too great your immune protection fails and you develop an illness.

No one is immune from the effects of stress; for example, children as yet unborn sometimes develop peptic ulcers. But whatever the variety and the timing of your stress, your reaction to it is determined by your constitution, and depends on how your genes instruct you to react. Whatever your reaction, a specific pattern of Vata-Pitta-Kapha derangement must develop in order for a specific disease to manifest. Whatever the pattern of this derangement, it is due fundamentally to weakness of Ojas and immunity.

Prana, Tejas and Ojas

Prana is the life force, equivalent to the chi or ki in Oriental medicine. It strings body, mind and spirit together on a single strand of breath, like pearls on a thread, and causes them to live, to act together as a single organism. Tejas is the force of transmutation, which permits body, mind and spirit to influence one another in spite of their different planes of existence. Ojas is the subtlest manifestation of the force of immunity, which is your individuality, the glue which cements these

123

pieces together and integrates your being. Prana, Tejas and Ojas unite body, mind and spirit.

Vata, Pitta and Kapha, the Three Doshas, are the gross manifestations of Prana, Tejas and Ojas, which are not Doshas at all. Vata is the more unstable form of Prana, Pitta the more reactive form of Tejas, and Kapha the more inert form of Ojas. When physical, mental and spiritual digestion are at their peak Vata, Pitta and Kapha are produced from Prana, Tejas and Ojas in quantities just sufficient to perform necessary bodily functions. Poor digestion allows greater production of these reactive by-products, reducing thereby the amount of the essential forces which the organism has available to it. Increased Vata, Pitta and Kapha production also requires increased excretion, and further energy loss.

We obtain Prana from our atmosphere and from our food. Breathing recharges Prana immediately. Prana is not oxygen, any more than Kapha is mucus or Pitta is bile. Prana is the life force; oxygen is one of its carrier substances. Food and water also carry Prana. While most of our nutrients are absorbed into the circulation from the small intestine, Prana is absorbed from the colon. Modern research shows that substances called volatile fatty acids are absorbed from the colon into the circulation and can act as a significant energy source for the system. These volatile fatty acids, like oxygen, are carriers of Prana. The health of our lungs and colons determines how much Prana we can absorb, and thus how alive we feel.

When the lungs or the large intestine function inefficiently, our bodies absorb Prana inefficiently, and Vata is generated in increased amounts. Vata and Prana are alike, both being airy, intense, expansive and subtle, but Vata is not inherently balancing and nutritive, as is Prana. Unless Vata is regularly excreted from the system it causes disease. Although disturbed Vata can affect any Dhatu it shows special affinity for Bone. The health of Bone is thus intimately tied to the health of the lungs and the colon. Hence Vimalananda's advice to keep the body (the bones) moving, the bowels (the colon) moving, and the breath (the lungs) moving.

Pathologies in the lungs, bones and large intestine are often related. For example, women who smoke lose more calcium from their bones because of the effect of carbon monoxide in the smoke on blood chemistry. Likewise, balancing one of these organs can benefit the others. Dry ginger mixed with jaggery (solidified sugar cane juice) improves the flow of urine and feces and when it is given to patients of upper respiratory congestion may relieve this congestion by relieving congestion in the colon. Sometimes medicated enemas are administered to control an attack of asthma.

Tejas is Fire. Just as a bellows inflames a hearthfire, Prana inflames Tejas. When the mind is stable and discrimination is strong, Tejas burns cleanly and purely and is transferred efficiently to the body. When the mind is affected by motion or inertia, or discrimination is agitated by memory or swamped by emotion, Tejas is perverted, and its transfer into the body produces greater amounts of Pitta. Since consciousness is strongly influenced by chemical toxins transported by blood, the ability of Tejas to properly nourish the physical digestion depends on blood, on the liver and spleen, which control blood, and on the brain.

Ojas is the medium through which the force of Tejas is transmitted. Both physical and mental digestion can be strong only when Ojas is strong. Ojas and Kapha are closely related. When there is good digestion of food and other sensory impressions, Ojas is efficiently produced. Weakened digestion causes increased Kapha production, and promotes production of Ama.

Ojas is a substance, unlike Tejas and Prana, which means it can be produced, collected, and stored. Anything which increases Vata decreases Ojas, including dry or stale food, excessive exposure to wind and sun, worry, fear, sorrow, old age, fasting from sleep, and excessive loss of any body tissue. Loss of Shukra, which nourishes Ojas directly, is more detrimental than loss of other tissues. This is one reason why sexual restraint is recommended in Ayurveda.

Ama is the sinister counterpart Ojas. Ojas is a living force which protects the integrity of the individual. Ama is a living force in the sense that it is a rich broth of nutrients for any alien invaders like bacteria, viruses, and cancer cells who might choose to colonize the system.

When Ojas is strong Tejas can properly digest and assimilate food and nourish all the Dhatus, which strengthens Ahamkara and your identity. A strong central identity will not allow either Ama or intruders to remain in the system. Weak Ojas interferes with the transmission of Tejas, which weakens the digestion and encourages production of Ama. Ama is useful nutrition only for intruders, so this weakens both the Dhatus and Ahamkara. A weak Ahamkara in turn encourages alien identities to flourish in the muck of Ama, just as a weak government encourages the proliferation of lawlessness.

Ojas is the foundation of your physical immunity, and produces your aura. Your aura is your first line of defense against intrusions from the outside. It is a buffer against all the negativity which is consciously and unconsciously projected against us each day. Weak Ojas allows more negativity to seep through the aura barrier, increasing internal disharmony. The weaker your aura, the less stress you can simply shrug off and ignore.

Indigestion

Indigestion is the base of all physical diseases, the condition from which all other conditions arise. In a sense indigestion, the inability of an individual to digest any physical, mental or emotional input, is the sole disease of living beings. It usually begins in the mind as a "crime against wisdom," and is projected from the mind into the physical body.

All disease results from a combination of physical, mental and spiritual causes. Some diseases like ulcerative colitis are mainly due to mental influences; others like the common cold are mainly physical. Patients who suffer from both a mental and a physical disease, such as schizophrenia and asthma, usually find that the physical problem gets worse whenever the mental disorder goes into remission, and vice versa. Ultimately all diseases are mental; all are caused by willfulness, that perversion of intellect and common sense which makes us do what we are not supposed to do. This willful perversity is Prajnaparadha, "crime against wisdom."

For example, suppose you are a VK person living in northern Minnesota. It is the middle of the night in the middle of winter and a blizzard is blowing outside. You are suddenly struck by a craving for ice cream. You know that ice cream is cold, wet, sticky, heavy and Kapha-producing, and that both night and winter are Kapha times, and that your constitution has Kapha in it. You know that if you eat the ice cream you are begging to increase Kapha, but you do it anyway, and the next morning your system is thoroughly clogged with Kapha. This is the punishment for a "crime against wisdom."

Transcontinental airplane flight is a stress to anyone regardless of constitution. You can travel coast to coast in about six hours, crossing three time zones in the process. Your consciousness arrives at your destination in six hours, and accompanies you off the plane. Your body, however, does not really arrive until three days later, since it takes about a day for it to recover from each time zone you cross. If you take the time to rest and recuperate from your journey you can adapt easily to your new location.

Your mind, however, hates to remain still, and does not like to permit the body to remain still. It is convinced that its balance is contingent on getting pending work out of the way as quickly as possible. Intercontinental air travel is a stress; so is trying to go to work as soon as you land. Your mind's impatience with your body over its jetlag strain further impedes the adaptation process. If your mind gets its way, and you try to go about business as usual, there is a good chance that your body will sulk, and will express its displeasure by becoming ill. Nature thus extracts from you the penalty for this "crime against wisdom."

The mind's physiology parallels that of the body. Like the physical Five Great Elements the mind has its own Five Elements:

> Stability, the mental equivalent of Earth;
> Emotion, the mental equivalent of Water;
> Discrimination, the mental equivalent of Fire;

Memory, the mental equivalent of Air; and
Emptiness, the mental equivalent of Ether.

Emptiness of mind is that which permits the other states of mind to manifest. Discrimination is the mind's digestion, which determines whether or not a course of action is appropriate for the well-being of the organism. As long as your power of discrimination functions normally you will turn away from committing "crimes against wisdom." Because your discrimination is often conditioned by the condition of your mind, mental instability weakens your ability to discriminate, just as disturbance of Vata, Pitta and Kapha affect the physical body's digestive capacity. Weak discrimination encourages the formation of mental Ama (abnormal perceptions), just as weak digestion allows physical Ama (toxic wastes) to be produced.

Vata, Pitta and Kapha are in charge of uniting the Five Great Physical Elements together in the body. Sattva, Rajas and Tamas perform the same function for the mind. Healthful, simple, well-digested food and healthful, simple habits promote Sattva. Intense, stimulating foods and intense activities like sex promote Rajas. Stale, putrid food and dulling activities like sleep promote Tamas. Rajas and Tamas are the Doshas of the mind. They are needed in small quantities, but cause disease when they accumulate to excess.

Good physical digestion is associated with these signs:

1. You feel no discomfort after ingesting your desired quantity of food.
2. After eating you do not belch gas which has the same odor and taste as the food you ate.
3. Your stomach does not feel full for an unusual length of time after your meal.
4. No symptoms are produced as the food passes through your small intestine and colon; you should not even be aware of this stage of digestion.
5. You excrete your feces at your habitual time. It must be of the proper consistency and should have no blood, mucus or undigested food in it, nor should it be offensive in odor.
6. After digestion your physical desire for food returns at the usual hour. (A mental desire for gratification of the tongue does not count.)

If any of the above is lacking, physical indigestion is present.

Good mental digestion is associated with these signs:

1. You feel no mental discomfort after ingesting your desired quantity of sense objects.
2. Your mind does not feel full and jaded afterwards.
3. No untoward emotions are produced during the period of time

you are processing this new information.

4. You can effortlessly and accurately retrieve your experience from memory and be able to communicate it if need be.

5. Your sleep after indulgence is sound and enjoyable, without disturbing dreams (which are indicative of mental Ama).

6. Desire for further sensory gratification arises after an appropriate period of time.

If any of the above is lacking, mental indigestion is present.

Physical indigestion can cause mental indigestion, and vice versa, but most often the two exist together. Because the body is much easier to control than the mind, Ayurveda believes that it is best to first purify and balance the body as much as possible and then turn to working with the mind, so that the harmonized body can exert a harmonizing effect on the mind.

Physical indigestion is basically of three types: that caused by Vata, that caused by Pitta, and that caused by Kapha. Any one of these Doshas can cause the body to lose its ability to process food, but each does it in a different way. We can know by the symptoms produced which Dosha is predominantly disturbed.

Vata-caused indigestion mainly affects the large intestine. Constipation alternates with loose stools, and there is usually copious intestinal gas, but all symptoms are variable. For a few days digestion improves, and then for no apparent reason the old symptoms return. The situation is so ever-changing that the individual does not know what to eat or when to eat to produce the intermittent spells of good digestion.

Pitta-caused indigestion affects mainly the small intestine, and usually causes loose stools. Burning sensations are common, such as heartburn or anal burning after defecation. The patient may crave hot spicy food, which only worsens the condition.

Kapha-caused indigestion affects mainly the stomach. The sufferer usually feels no desire for food at all, and usually has heaviness in the upper abdomen, watering of the mouth, and heaviness in the limbs. Constipation is common.

Kapha is most at home in the stomach, Pitta in the small intestine, and Vata in the colon. If indigestion is allowed to continue untreated one or more of these Doshas will increase greatly, leave its home organ and begin to circulate in the system searching for a weak area in which it can locate and cause a disease. Untreated indigestion thus results in acute diseases like colds, fevers, coughs, influenza, diarrhea, peptic ulcer, and so on. All these diseases are methods Nature uses to purify your organism when your being cannot "digest" life's experiences and instead allows physical and mental filth to collect inside you.

No matter how efficiently you treat an acute disease, your effort will be wasted unless you also address the underlying indigestion. Unless you eliminate this root, other diseases will later sprout from it. Treatment should begin with the uprooting of the root cause of the disease, and should then concern itself with any specific manifestations. Life-threatening situations require emergency attention, true, but once the crisis passes the indigestion remains to be tackled.

Ayurvedic Treatment

A Yogi named Chaitanyananda lived about 200 miles from Bombay until his death not long ago. His cures of serious diseases, extending even to the first stages of cancer, were well documented, and people flocked from all over India to receive treatment at his hands.

He would welcome with profuse greetings anyone who came to him, to create in them a false sense of security. While they rested he would go into the jungle to collect a certain herb whose juice was then administered to the unsuspecting patient. About fifteen minutes later the poor sufferer would begin to vomit and purge. This vigorous purification lasted for up to three hours. After the nausea and diarrhea died down, the patient would be served split mung beans and rice cooked together into the preparation known as khichadi. Into this porridge Chaitanyananda would add a mixture of mineral and metallic oxides in a specific proportion according to the nature of the disease. After repeating this process for thirty days, the patient was clean from top to bottom, and the disease had disappeared.

Chaitanyananda never studied classical Ayurveda in a college, but his treatment followed Ayurvedic lines:

Removal of the cause.

Purification to eliminate excess Doshas.

Balancing the Doshas and rekindling the digestive fire.

Rejuvenation to rebuild the organism.

Any therapy which does not follow these steps is not Ayurvedic, nor is it likely to be permanently effective, because it fails to balance the Doshas. Even when your mind is unbalanced, that imbalance is either due to Dosha imbalance or is being made worse by it.

Faith was also an important ingredient in Chaitanyananda's cures. People came to him expecting relief because they had heard tales of all those whom he had helped, and this faith helped cure them. Remember that one symptom of diseased Rasa Dhatu is "lack of faith." Faith is the single most important aspect of cure because it enhances Ahamkara's ability to self-identify with the body, and actively works to strengthen Rasa Dhatu, which then nourishes the other Dhatus and Ojas too. Vimalananda always said that there are only two ways to cure a disease. You can have faith in another being—a physician, a deity, your grandmother, or anyone else—and putting yourself entirely in his or her hands allow that person to direct the force of your faith. Otherwise you must have faith in yourself, in your own powers of self-healing, and heal yourself directly.

If you have no Chaitanyananda to force you to become healthy, you are responsible for curing yourself. You must decide with all parts of your being that you are tired of being imbalanced and that you are prepared to undergo whatever discipline may be necessary to heal yourself. Until you can say to yourself sincerely that you are ready to change your ways healing cannot occur. A firm decision to heal yourself only happens when your mind is ready to admit to willfulness and "crimes against wisdom," when it is willing to admit to its deviousness in blaming the body for its own excesses. When your mind is truly contrite, and willing to forgive itself for falling ill, it is sure to cooperate with your body to do the job right.

Hopelessness or helplessness is dangerous because it deprives your immune system of support from Ahamkara. If your mind decides that it is fed up with any body part, that body part is likely to lose its immunity and become quickly devitalized. Be angry, be hostile, experience any emotion which wants to come out, but never fall prey to hopelessness if you want to be cured.

Moreover, you have to want everyone to be healthy if you want to become healthy. Nature's Law is that you get back whatever you put out, so you will get health only if your activities and attitudes promote, or at least do not interfere with, the health of those around you. Health is a lot like disease: it is contagious, and can be passed from one person to another over and over again.

The discussions below do not purport to be a guide to self-treatment of serious diseases. They merely outline some aspects of the Ayurvedic management of certain conditions. You should always seek expert professional guidance for any serious disorder.

Elimination of Ama

When your tongue is coated, your feces are foul, and your urine is turbid, Ama is present in your digestive tract and must be first removed before anything else is done. The best way to do this is to do nothing: allow the body to expel the Ama itself by fasting.

Fasting is the first and best of all medicines. When possible you should fast for 24 to 48 hours on as little intake of anything as possible. If you are acutely ill, as with a fever, this should not be too difficult because you will probably not want anything. Brew up some weak tea of dried ginger (to 1 tsp. per quart of water boiled for 20 minutes) and sip it, just enough to prevent you from becoming dehydrated. Add a few drops of lemon juice if you like. As soon as your urine, feces, and tongue clear, your digestive tract is free of Ama and purification can proceed. When you are not acutely ill, 24 to 48 hours on weak ginger tea might seem like an eternity if you are a V or a P. You can use thin rice gruel in addition to provide your body with some substance while it works to empty itself of Ama.

Once the Ama is gone from your digestive tract, Vata, Pitta and Kapha must flow freely again. This is the province of the therapies known collectively as Panchakarma: emesis, purgation, enema, nasal medication, and bloodletting. Emesis, or therapeutic vomiting, is the best way to improve flow when Kapha congestion has been the main cause of your disease. Purgation is meant to eliminate Pitta congestion, and enema controls Vata. Nasal medication works on Doshas accumulated in the head, and bloodletting purifies the Blood directly.

Ayurveda regards medicated enema as the most important purification method of all, because of the importance of the large intestine in health and disease. For example, the AIDS virus apparently first colonizes the colon and proliferates there before it floods the system. It can do so only if the colon is full of Ama to encourage it to grow. Medicated enemas eliminate pathogenic Ama and facilitate the absorption of Prana.

Your system must be well prepared before you undergo Panchakarma. Specifically:

1. *Determine which of your Doshas is most disturbed.* Usually your state of indigestion can tell you. Also consider your constitution, and this axiom:

> There is no *pain* without involvement of Vata.
> There is no *inflammation* without involvement of Pitta.
> There is no *pus formation* without involvement of Kapha.

Whenever there is intense pain, especially colicky or stabbing in nature, Vata is present. Whenever fever or inflammation predominate, as in an ulcer, Pitta is in excess. Whenever there is pus formation anywhere, even in the sputum as in bronchitis, Kapha is disturbed.

2. *Oil your body.* Whenever your body is full of Ama, the use of ordinary oils will create additional congestion, so use only castor oil. It can be applied externally to any areas which are painful or inflamed due to Ama, and used internally in the dose of 1 Tbsp. with a cup of strong tea made of powdered ginger to scrape Ama away from the tissues. When the body is relatively purified any oil can be used.

3. *Sweat.* Sweat is oil's partner in Vata control. Modern thermography shows that painful areas in the body where there is no inflammation are usually several degrees cooler than normal. This pain is the result of constricted blood vessels. One of the effects which pain-killing drugs show is a temporary restoration to normal temperatures

of these painful parts. Such cold may have a physical cause, or may be due to fear and other cold emotions.

Dry heat, like saunas or burying yourself under heavy blankets, should be used exclusively whenever there is any body obstruction due to Ama. Wet heat, like steam baths or hot tubs, can be used when there is little Ama. Normally, direct heat should not be applied to the eyes, heart and testicles.

4. *Purify*. Oil and heat "soften up" your system, and help mobilize all the Ama trapped in the Dhatus so that it can be excreted. The ancient texts use this analogy: A dried stick is so brittle that it breaks when it is bent, whereas if you first oil the stick well and then warm it gently it will regain its suppleness and again be able to bend without breaking. You must be careful to avoid "bending" your body with Panchakarma before adequately heating and oiling it, lest it be damaged.

Improperly administered purifications can cause side-effects, so use these measures with care. Purification must not be done during any extremes of climate—heat waves, cold snaps, flash floods, wind storms—and is forbidden to the very young, the very old, the very weak, and pregnant women.

In general:

When the patient is strong and the disease is weak use Panchakarma

When the patient is weak and the disease is strong, first balance the Doshas to weaken the disease and strengthen the patient before doing Panchakarma.

Panchakarma is not heroics. Like all other Ayurvedic therapies it emulates Nature's methods to assist Her in healing the individual. Here is an example: a few months ago I was helping a friend of mine perform some emergency maintenance on the brakes of his car. We were in Northern Ontario. It was early spring. Assuming that the work would be done quickly we postponed lunch.

We ended up spending almost five hours on the repairs. In the late afternoon, the Vata time of day, a chill wind blew up, which did nothing to improve our exasperation over the delay in the process. Eventually we got home, disappointed that we had missed our chance to go canoeing. Within half an hour of our arrival, my friend was down with a fever.

I knew it was due to Vata. It had arisen quickly, a characteristic of many Vata diseases. The causative factors were all Vata-producing: strenuous exertion leading to fatigue, cold wind, hunger, exasperation, late afternoon, and disappointment creating Bitterness. I told him to eat some fresh khichadi with ghee, to replenish the nutrients he had burned off by his exertion, and then to accompany me to the sauna, to allow its heat to control Vata's cold. Heat is not good for Pitta-type fevers, but may be appropriate for those due to Vata or Kapha.

He did as I suggested, and after a few moments in the heat became nauseated and had to leave to go vomit. I regarded this as a good sign: the khichadi had attracted the Vata to the stomach, the ghee had oiled his insides, and the sweat had facilitated Vata's movement. He returned to the sauna feeling much relieved, collected more heat, vomited once again, and went to bed. The next morning, after a good rest, he was as good as new. This procedure, which only helped Nature do what She wanted to do, would not work in every case, of course, but was just right for his.

Details of Panchakarma purification methods which can be done at home may be found in *Ayurveda: The Science of Self-Healing* by Dr. Vasant Lad.

TRIPHALA

Panchakarma is a wonderful thing, but it is only a beginning. If you have been mistreating your body for many years you have many layers of Ama to be removed. Each layer must be loosened before it can be dissolved off and expelled. Even if you could eliminate all Ama at once it would be unwise to do so because your organs of elimination might not be able to process all the toxins and you might seriously imbalance your system.

Besides, your organism has had these toxins in it so long that it has developed a metabolic equilibrium which involves them. It will resist all revolutionary changes, especially if there is a lot of fear-producing Vata in your constitution or condition, because it feels its metabolic rug being pulled from underneath it. Chaitanyananda avoided this problem by providing an environment of complete stability and security which the organism could use as a haven while its world was turned inside out. Unless you can retire from the world for at least six weeks, it is better to follow each spell of purification by weeks of balancing the Doshas and nourishing the Dhatus.

Panchakarma is a depletive procedure (called Apatarpana in Sanskrit), and all depletion tends to weaken Ahamkara. Unless Santarpana, or rebuilding the Dhatus, is adequate after Panchakarma your immunity is bound to weaken. For example, colonics may be beneficial for ridding the body of impurities, but if they are overused they will cause severe Vata disturbance because they deplete the system without offering anything in return. Since Vata produces fear, the system will actually hold onto any remaining Ama with increased tenacity. Your system must be confident; it must be willing to release its stored toxins if your purifications are to be successful. Slow and steady in purification is always best.

Excess in purification can actually drive Ama deeper into your tissues. For example, overuse of Hot, Pungent foods or herbs like garlic and cayenne, excessive exercise, and repression of emotions are equally likely to disturb the purification process as are more obvious violations of purification like restraint of natural urges, improper food combining and indulgence in stimulants like alcohol or caffeine. Although it may make you bored or impatient, you must be careful to purify at your system's preferred rate of speed.

Triphala can gradually, gently purify and rejuvenate your digestive tract, improving your ability to nourish your Dhatus. Triphala, which literally means "three fruits," is composed of three unique herbs: Amalaki, Haritaki and Bibhitaki. Amalaki's main Taste is Sour, but it also has Sweet, Bitter, Pungent, and Astringent secondary Tastes. Its Energy is Cold, and its Post-Digestive Effect is Sweet. It balances all Three Doshas but is best for controlling Pitta. It can improve the digestive fire through Sour without disturbing Pitta, thanks to Sweet and Cold. The fresh fruit is intensely Sour, but when you drink a glass of water after eating an Amalaki the water tastes as sweet as syrup.

One Amalaki the size of a plum contains 20 times the vitamin C of an orange. This vitamin C is in a heat-stable form and survives the cooking or drying processes used during the fruit's preparation. Amalaki is especially used for hyperacidity and for liver complaints. It is used in shampoos, and oil medicated with it improves the hair and brain. It is a superior rejuvenator; one of its Sanskrit names is "Wet-Nurse," in honor of the care with which it like sleep improves body and mind.

Haritaki's main Taste is Astringent, but it is also Sweet, Sour, Bitter, and Pungent secondarily. It has Hot Energy and Sweet Post-Digestive Effect. It balances all Three Doshas but is best for Vata because it can consolidate the body and mind with its Astringency while controlling Vata via Sweet and Hot. It scrapes old adherent Ama from the digestive tract and tones the colon.

Bibhitaki's main Taste is also Astringent, with secondary Sweet, Bitter and Pungent, Hot Energy, and Sweet Post-digestive Effect. It balances all Three Doshas but is best for Kapha in spite of being Sweet because it is Astringent and Hot. It purifies all body fluids and is especially good in asthma and hiccoughs.

Triphala is the Ayurvedic panacea. You can use it to wash your hair or body, or as a laxative, purgative, or emetic, or in an enema. Its decoction can be used as eye, nose, or ear drops, or for gargling. It scrapes toxins from body tissues, and causes Doshas which have left their proper locations—stomach, small intestine, and colon—to return there. Because of its powerful ability to purify it is also used to detoxify substances like metals before they are prepared into medicines. Triphala is harmless, but very toxic persons sometimes react if they use too large a dose because it mobilizes their stored toxins faster than their weakened systems can process them.

The best way to use Triphala powder for gradual purification and re-generation of the digestive tract is to stir 1 tsp. into a glass of pure water and let it sit overnight. The next morning you should drink the water without stirring, allowing the sediment to remain on the bottom. You then refill the glass, stir vigorously, let it sit all day long, and drink it again at night without stirring. Then discard the dregs and stir a fresh teaspoonful into a fresh glass of water for the next day.

If this is too laxative a dose or causes some reaction, drink only one glass daily. Let the refilled glass stand all day and all night, drink it the next morning, and after discarding the remains prepare a fresh mixture for the next morning. In this way 1 tsp. will last you for two days. If this still causes a reaction, reduce the amount to 1/2 tsp. You should continue this routine for three to six months for maximum benefit.

FASTING

Ayurveda frowns on long-term fasting because the sense of depriva-tion created by a long fast encourages you to follow it with a long spell of indulgence to rebuild Ahamkara's confidence. I knew a Westerner in India who had decided to fast his way to enlightenment. He was an ex-treme example of the V constitution so I knew it would be dangerous and warned him pointedly about the possible perils. It was impossible to change his mind; he obstinately ignored all warnings. One day his starving, devitalized immune system landed him in the hospital, where doctors lanced a long abscess running all the way up his leg. The out-come of this adventure into higher consciousness? After his recovery he returned to North America and became a cook!

His obsession with food never left him, because his persistent fast-ing so starved his Dhatus that they eventually overwhelmed his resolve. This cycle of overrestriction followed by overgratification aggravates Vata in everyone who attempts it. It is better to fast regularly for a day once every week or two. The digestive organs need a day off as much as any human workers do, and it will not do to make them work over-time for months in a row without any rest and then give them a long enforced fasting vacation.

During an illness you should fast as long as you have no real desire for food. As long as you feel lighter, brighter and healthier without food, continue your fast. As soon as you begin to lose your energy and feel real hunger, consume well-cooked rice or barley gruel until that also fails to satisfy your appetite, and then switch to khichadi, the prepara-tion of rice and split mung beans whose recipe is given in the Appen-dix. It purifies and nourishes the Dhatus and is an ideal diet during prolonged therapy of any chronic disease because it relaxes and light-ens the mind while eliminating both mental and physical Ama.

Fasting is used as a purification only if Panchakarma cannot be done. Therefore, daily enemas and other such heroic procedures should form no part of your fast. If you do choose to fast for a prolonged period, you should get professional guidance if you have never fasted before. You may experience acute physical stress if your system begins to mobilize Ama faster than your organs of excretion can handle it.

You should also follow the restrictions applicable to your constitution. V people, for example, should never fast on water or any other severely restricted diet for more than a day or two. Absolute fasting for as little as a week can wreck metabolic balance which may have taken months to obtain.

V types should select a single food, like khichadi, on which they can live for a month or more at a time. P people can fast on liquids like fruit or vegetable juices or on raw fruits and vegetables, but not on water alone. They should not skimp on quantity. K people alone may indulge in a prolonged water fast if they so desire. Otherwise, they may use raw juices. K people especially need regular weekly fasting to maintain strong digestion.

V people may fast once weekly or bi-monthly on liquids other than water alone. Some Vs like lemon juice and honey in pure water; others enjoy juices, and those who are not allergic to dairy may prefer milk, fresh whey, or yogurt blended with water. None of these should be refrigerator cold. Ps should use diluted fruit juices, like grape, prune or pomegranate, or Bitter or Astringent vegetable juices like cucumber. They should avoid all Sour juices. K types should avoid both intensely Sweet and Sour juices.

Balancing the Doshas

Whether or not you have used Panchakarma for purification, you must balance your imbalanced Doshas.

If you have a V constitution, or if your indigestion and Ama formation were due to Vata, you may use:

Dry ginger, fennel, or dill to digest Ama.

Lemon, lime or grapefruit for the Sour Taste, rock salt for the Salty Taste, and ginger or garlic for the Pungent Taste to rekindle your digestion. Medicinal wines are excellent for the V digestive fire.

Light, well-cooked food and warm liquids, especially with ginger added.

Mild exercise, especially simple Yoga stretches; regular sunbathing; and indirect ventilation, since strong winds increase Vata.

If Pitta caused your problem, you may use:

Fennel to digest Ama. You may use dry ginger if it is not too intense for you.

Psyllium seed husks, Triphala, or any Bitter herb like gentian to re-kindle your digestion.

Light or raw foods and juices with cold coriander or sandalwood tea.

Strolling in the open air, especially near flowing water; moderate sunbathing, early or late in the day; and regular exposure to wind to help dry Pitta.

If Kapha caused your problem, you may use:

Dry ginger, black pepper, or cumin to digest Ama.

Any Bitter or Pungent herbs like garlic or black pepper to enkindle the digestive fire.

Small quantities of food, especially roasted, with as little liquid as possible; tea of dry ginger is best.

Vigorous exercise; extensive sunbathing, well-wrapped if need be to encourage sweating; and windbathing, well-wrapped to preserve body heat.

Psyllium seed husks, known as isabgol or flea-seed husks in India, are an excellent way to purify the intestines. If they are being used to absorb excess water from the body, they should be taken dry; otherwise they should first be soaked in some liquid to prevent them from causing constipation and congestion. If you are not allergic to dairy, psyllium husks should be soaked in milk to relieve constipation, and in a blend of yogurt and water to relieve loose stools.

Because it is heavy for digestion, regular use of psyllium over a long period of time weakens the digestive fire in V and K types. This can be prevented by consuming an ounce of a medicinal wine diluted with an ounce of water at the same time that you take the psyllium. Since Ayurvedic medicinal wines are not readily available, an ounce of organic additive-free wine diluted with an ounce of water, or half a cup of tea made of dry ginger, may be used instead.

Even after you quit using medicines your dietary control must continue and you must restrict your normal habits of indulgence for at least six weeks. The texts list eight common practices which can recreate a disease in those who are healing:

Excessive and forceful talking; Travelling, especially long distance; Excessive walking; Continual sitting or lying in one position; Overeating leading to indigestion; Inappropriate diet with improper food combining; Sleeping during the day (except in summer); and Any kind of sexual activity.

Mental Medication

Balancing Vata is sure to reduce fear but cannot eliminate it entirely, especially if an individual has a V constitution, whose very genes possess the potential to create fear. Fear is always intensified and worsened by worry, so a V person should be kept occupied and never be given time to worry. Meditation is the best occupation, the only direct way to eliminate fear. Exercise or a hobby may be useful, as long as it can induce the individual to concentrate on it. Vs must guard against addiction, however, which can develop to any kind of active recreation. Passive pursuits, like listening to music or even enjoying spectator sports, are also addictive, but their passive nature is less likely to exhaust a V.

Likewise, anger can only be reduced, not eliminated, in a P individual, who has anger-creating genes. Impatience, which produces anger or jealousy, is the key disturbance in the P individual. Since it usually occurs when the mind is idle, the P mind should always have something to work on. Mere pastimes will not suffice, as they may for Vata, because Pitta needs problems to gnaw on, "digest" and solve little by little. Difficult problems are good because Ps will usually stay with a project until it is finished, but not a moment longer. Any sort of complicated project which is beneficial to the individual will do.

K people have complacency in their genes. Treatment of Kapha-caused indigestion can only control it, not eliminate it. Complacency may manifest as greed to consume and possess whatever one can obtain, or it may indicate a lackadaisical attitude toward health. The Earth in Kapha tends to set K people stubbornly in their ways. Vigorous motivation, by self or others, is the only way to balance these traits. It is best to concentrate on one activity in the beginning. Though it may take quite a while, once a K individual becomes dedicated to self-improvement his or her inertial force will cause the progression to continue, though without periodic "booster" doses of motivation it may gradually slow to a halt again.

Our ability to act on our intentions is limited by our capacity to integrate them into ourselves. A Sattvic person, who has an abundance of mental equilibrium or Sattva, comprehends well and follows his or her path steadily and consistently, and progresses quickly. Rajasic people, who are full of the hyperactivity of Rajas, twist facts to fit their preconceptions, and convince themselves that they are progressing when they are in fact merely reinforcing Ahamkara's dependencies. Tamasic people, whose abundant inert Tamas guides their being, ignore clear evidence of the need to progress and dig in where they are in hope of remaining there.

Mental digestion predominates over physical digestion. If you bite off more than you can chew, be it a book you are writing or a cake you are eating, you do so because of weakness of Ahamkara. She is weak but believes herself to be strong, and tries to prove it with overambition. If your mind is relatively clear this self-delusion will be temporary, and you remove the "food" from your "mouth" before trying to chew it up.

If you tenaciously hold onto your "food" and try determinedly to chew it up you will be chewing up more than you can swallow. You can still spit out the "food" whenever you admit to your self-deception, but the longer you hold onto it the more Ahamkara invests in displaying to the world that she can do everything she sets out to do. Allowing Ahamkara's investment in her assumed persona to regulate your life causes you to swallow more than you can digest.

At this stage you can prevent undigested experience from entering your system by "vomiting" it: making a clean breast of the affair and admitting to a "crime against wisdom." If you fail to do this physical or mental Ama is created and absorbed into your system, and some disease or another becomes inevitable.

A friend of mine recently opened a school for herbal studies, and permitted his ambition to overwhelm his mental digestion. He enrolled fifteen students, both because he needed their fees to break even and because he felt he was strong enough to teach them all adequately. As the term progressed he found himself overwhelmed by the needs of these fifteen diverse individuals and began to overwork. His ability to follow through could not keep pace with his intentions. In his enthusiasm to empower others by transferring his knowledge to them he was ruining his own health.

The stress of continuously having to adapt to fifteen different Ahamkaras depressed his digestion and created mental Ama. Because he would not at first admit to himself that he had overextended his limits he buried that Ama inside himself. For self-protection his mind projected the imbalance into his body. When last we met he was complaining of symptoms which suggested a disturbed gall bladder.

His diet was appropriate for his constitution, and the season was not Pitta-aggravating, so I knew his problems were mainly based in his mind. As we conversed he himself made the connection between imperfect mental digestion and weakness of a physical digestive organ, and realized that he needed to eliminate the indigestible situation which was causing his problem. He could do this by decreasing his student load, or by enlisting assistance to help him with it. His recognition of the problem ensured that he would be able to solve it.

Management of mental disorders involves essentially the same steps outlined for physical treatment. When poor mental digestion has created many untoward emotions and the accumulation of those emotions eventually distorts the self-image and the ability to function efficiently, removal of the cause is the first requisite. Then the mind must be purified. A mind filled with anger releases the anger fairly easily, and thus purifies itself somewhat, but a mind filled with fear holds onto its' fear tenaciously and releases it only after consistent application of mental heat and oil, which is Sneha, sincere affection. Mental inertia requires strenuous stimulation to induce it to purify.

Of course, if the individual's mind is weak and the disorder is strong purification is unwise, as it will further weaken the mind. Then balancing of Rajas and Tamas with the power of Sattva is first essential. Mental rejuvenation is indicated in all cases.

When the mind is filled with Ama created from unsatisfactory interpersonal relationships, fasting from cravings is a must. There is even a mental Triphala to help scrape away the old Ama of selfish atachments. It is called Kirtana, the devotional singing of God's name. Even if you don't believe in a God with form, you can select a name which represents whatever you do believe in, and repeat it with devotion, allowing that force to enter and heal you.

Kirtana is also the best rejuvenator, because it helps us rectify our relationship with Nature. The true meaning of Yoga is union with the divine, and an attitude of sincere request for divine assistance is the royal road to real Yoga.

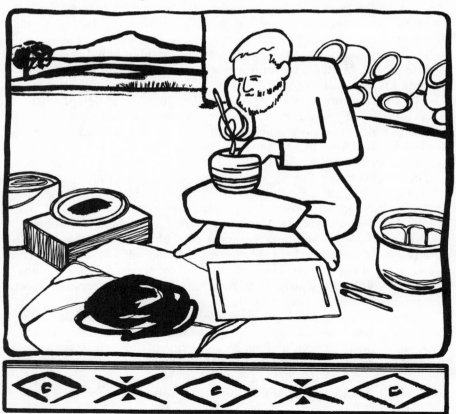

Yukti

The word "Yukti" is derived from the same root as the word Yoga. Yukti is defined in Sanskrit as "bahu-karana-yoga-ja": created from the union of many causes. A clay pot, for example, is created by Yukti. It is a union of clay, water, a wheel, a stick to form the pot, a kiln to fire it, fuel for the kiln, and a potter to oversee the entire process.

Health is produced by Yukti. One person's cancer may disappear after treatment with powerful medicines; another's may recede after visualizations alone; a third's may respond exclusively to diet. Cure depends on a therapy which may be more or less complex, a patient who must have faith in something, individuals who will administer the therapies to the patient, and a director to oversee. Above all, there must be a competent director. It may be the patient himself or herself, but there must be someone who knows what to do and when it needs to be done. It is said that even if the remedy is insufficient, the assistants are incompetent, and the patient is recalcitrant, a skillful therapist can still provide relief, using the principle of Yukti to combine removal of the cause, purification, balancing and rejuvenation into one harmonious whole therapy.

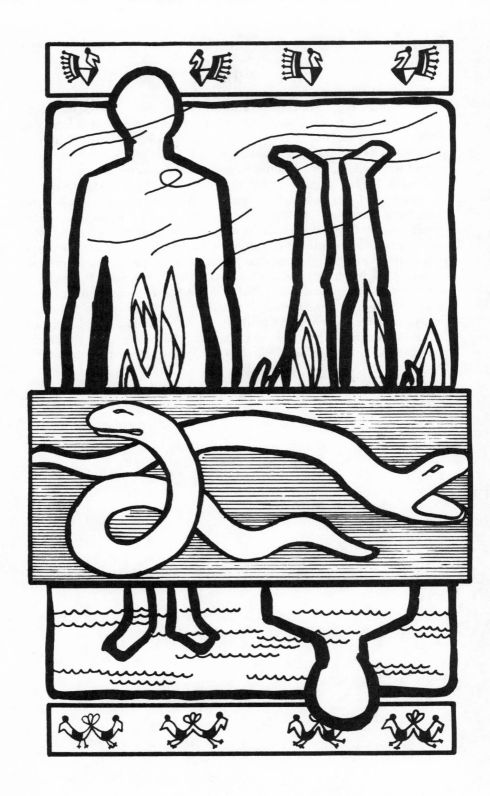

Chapter Seven

Disease

Without Yukti, the adept combination of attitude and activity to harmonize the individual, indigestion becomes chronic, and mutates into new forms. Chronic indigestion weakens the immune system, which reacts first with allergy, then with auto-immune disease, and finally with conditions in which immunity collapses altogether, like cancer or AIDS. Weakness of Ahamkara's self-identification with the body is the root cause of all such conditions.

Allergy

An antigen is anything, usually but not always a protein, which can be recognized as being foreign to the organism. Ama is a general term for antigenic material. Every piece of improperly digested food which gets absorbed into your system is Ama. Antibodies are special proteins created by some of your white blood cells which are made to order in response to exposure to specific antigens. The antibodies bind tightly to the antigens, and if your immune system is healthy it completes its policing job by sweeping the antibody-antigen complexes from the body.

Your immune system can identify the source of each sort of Ama: cheese Ama, pork Ama, peanut Ama, and so on. When you are exposed over and over again to the same Ama, more and more antibodies are produced as your system steels itself against the next wave of invaders. If you know you do not digest peanuts well, and yet you persistently, perversely consume them, those imperfectly digested peanuts persistently form Ama. Eventually so much peanut Ama accumulates in you that whenever a peanut touches your tongue your immune police sound an alarm, assuming that it too will be improperly digested. When the immune reaction is so pronounced that you are made aware of it by some bodily or mental symptom caused as a side-effect of the internal combat, you have an allergy.

Humans can become allergic to almost anything. One source has estimated that 30% of the American populace has some degree of food allergy. Some people are allergic to mold, others to hydrocarbons and petrochemicals, still others to cat or dog hair. Some people break out into hives when they are exposed to sudden cold. There is even a condition called exercise-induced anaphylaxis in which strenuous exertion produces an allergic reaction which can be life-threatening. This, like the allergy to cold, is probably due to the toxic state of the organism, and not to a specific allergy to aerobics. The sudden stress of the activity causes toxins to be mobilized from their tissue storage sites and flood the circulation.

Almost any symptom can be caused in an allergic reaction. While acute disease with fever and/or pus is not likely to be allergic, nor are unilateral conditions (pains, swellings, and the like on one side of the body only), the tendency to bilateral pains and swellings and to recurrent, repeated infections which might have pus and fever, like "chronic colds" and infections of the tonsils and ears, is often allergic.

Allergies occur in a hypersensitive organism. While specific allergies may respond to specific desensitization techniques, management of the allergic state involves reducing this hypersensitivity. Vata and Pitta are the principal Doshas involved in allergy, because it is their mutual intensity which oversensitizes the organism.

Allergies can be of many different types. Some only occur if you take the allergen often enough, since otherwise antibody levels never build up high enough to induce a noticeable reaction. Others occur every time you consume a substance. The most insidious are the addictive allergies. As long as you take the substance you are allergic to, you feel fine; as soon as you quit, you start to feel withdrawal symptoms.

This can be tested by examining your cravings carefully. Suppose you like to eat chocolate. If you crave it only occasionally, and feel satisfied after a small piece, your body probably created that craving in you for some specific purpose. Perhaps it needed to balance itself out with the help of some factor which is found in chocolate. If however you have to have chocolate every day or you feel out of sorts, or if you eat a small piece of chocolate and then suddenly experience an almost uncontrollable craving to consume all the chocolates in the box, then you very likely have an addictive allergy to the chocolate. All addictions, even to the most virulent drugs, probably become allergic in nature with time.

The allergic tendency develops early in life, and is strongly influenced by prakruti. V and P types are much more commonly affected by allergy than are Ks. Even modern allergists note that most of their patients of food allergy are blond-haired and blue-eyed, whom we can recognize as P, PV or PK types.

In addition, after conception when the child is growing in the womb the mother sends some of her immune protection to her fetus across the placenta in the form of antibodies. If she is very toxic, she may send too many antibodies, or she may even transmit antigens circulating in her blood to her fetus. Immune reactions may begin in the baby's body even before birth. After birth, the mother's breast milk is supposed to provide passive immunity to the child. If it also carries antigenic material to the baby, or if the child is not breast-fed long enough, its immunity will suffer.

The nature of the allergens to which you are exposed is also important. For example, allergy to alcohol, which probably influences the development of both hangovers and alcoholism, may actually begin as allergy to the grain used in the fermentation process. Likewise, milk allergy may develop from lactose intolerance, or it may begin as allergy to the penicillin which is given to the cows as a disease preventative and then progress to allergy to the milk itself. Pork allergy may begin as tetracycline sensitivity. Mass-produced chickens are fed many different drugs, all of which might sensitize the body against the chicken.

Intestinal toxemia is also involved in the development of allergy. Pollution in the large intestine permits the irritating chemicals produced by improper digestion to be absorbed into your system and carried via your circulation to other parts of your body. All of this is Ama, which sets up reactions wherever it goes. These internal pollutants inflame the membrane lining the large intestine and reduce mobility, causing the body to absorb toxins which otherwise would be excreted. For example, improper digestion of the amino acid tyrosine produces the corrosive chemical phenol. One drop of pure phenol can burn a hole in your external skin; imagine its effect, even in diluted form, on the internal skin lining the digestive tract.

Intestinal toxemia adversely affects your brain as well. Since your brain's consciousness is chemically based, each toxin alters it. Proper digestion of the amino acid tryptophan yields serotonin, the brain's "mellow chemical" which keeps us cool, calm and collected. Improper digestion of tryptophan produces indole and skatole, the chemicals which give feces its offensive odor. They agitate and disturb the brain. Swallowing tablets of L-tryptophan may increase serotonin and temporarily calm the brain, but if it is improperly digested the long-term result will be greater agitation, thanks to increased indole and skatole.

Abnormal processes also produce substances like octopamine which are called "false neurotransmitters." They can replace the normal neurotransmitters, whose job is to accurately transfer messages across the brain, leaving the consciousness further scattered and disorganized, unable to properly monitor or maintain the organism's immune defenses.

Just as Ama created from improper digestion of food can disturb the consciousness and agitate the emotions, disturbed emotions can weaken the digestion and create Ama, which then incites the immune system to react against it. Deeply suppressed emotions amplify the allergic reaction, as the mind feels threatened by its inability to express itself and takes out its frustrations on the substances which are invading it. A complete physical housecleaning would remedy the situation, but a deeply agitated mind will usually try to make use of every opportunity for sensory indulgence. The continuous presence of Ama in the system creates a condition of permanent immune alert, an allergic state.

Rheumatic Disease

Persistent allergies eventually develop into more serious conditions. Ama becomes so tightly wedged into you that some of your own tissues are destroyed by immune reactions. These dead cells are foreign bodies, an internally-derived variety of Ama, and the immune system engulfs and devours them just as it would attack any other intruders. Eventually your immune cells acquire a cannibalistic taste for living tissue of the type which it has been scavenging. This is an "auto-immune" reaction.

Auto-immune disease has been described as conditioned, or limited, malignancy. Since the ageing process is mediated by auto-immune processes, and since all of us die of old age if no other disease claims us earlier, auto-immunity must be eliminated before rejuvenation becomes possible.

Rheumatic disease provides a good example of an auto-immune condition which can often be successfully managed by an Ayurvedic approach. The rheumatic diseases—rheumatic fever, rheumatism, and rheumatoid arthritis—are conditions in which the body is filled with "rheum," a form of Ama. About 10% of all patients who see a doctor have some rheumatic disease, an indication of how deeply ill the general public has become. Like rheumatic fever, rheumatoid arthritis can affect the heart, and can actually kill. It is a serious, life-threatening condition.

Rheumatoid arthritis is a generalized systemic disease which can occur at any age, though it is less common in children and teenagers than it is in adults. Younger people are more prone to rheumatic fever, which is still common in some less developed countries and is basically an acute form of the same disease process. On the average, rheumatoid arthritis first appears around age forty. There is a hereditary tendency involved, and women are affected three to five times as often as men are. While it affects people in all parts of the world it is significantly more severe in cold, damp climates, which promote Kapha congestion and Ama accumulation.

Rheumatoid arthritis is called Ama-Vata in Sanskrit, which means that it occurs when Vata circulates Ama all throughout the body. The most important initiating cause seems to be improper diet, which creates Ama. Other causes include exhaustion due to overwork, excessive exercise, frequent sex, intense worry, and emotional disturbances such as grief. Exhaustion and strong emotion aggravate Vata; they make rheumatoid arthritis worse and can sometimes initiate it. Overuse of intoxicants, especially alcohol, simultaneously disturb Vata and create Ama.

The sticky, opaque, offensive sludge which is Ama can be found in the joints of every sufferer of rheumatoid arthritis. This is one sure way to distinguish rheumatoid arthritis from osteoarthritis, which is a localized manifestation of the ageing process. If synovial fluid, that sticky, highly viscous lubricant which lubricates our joints, is withdrawn from a osteoarthritic joint it will be nearly normal, but in rheumatoid or bacterial arthritis the fluid loses its ability to lubricate, becomes turbid, contains cells of many types in large numbers, and even clots on standing. Healthy synovial fluid never clots.

Synovial fluid is one of the body's repositories of the force of Kapha. Kapha and Ama are much alike in quality, so it is not surprising that Ama should have affinity for the joints. This Ama originates mainly in the colon, where improper fat metabolism creates a variety of Ama which shows a special affinity for the bones and joints. Since the membrane lining the colon is intimately connected with the nutrition of cartilage and bone, this Ama swiftly reaches its preferred location and deposits itself. The immune system sweeps in to attack, and the disease is created. If allowed to continue unchecked the inflammation becomes chronic and destroys the joint, which causes nearby muscles to atrophy. All this happens because of undigested material in the colon.

Menstrual irregularities predispose women to rheumatoid arthritis. Women are physically more fortunate then men, because each month their Blood is purified by the menstrual flow. During the first part of the month the body provides the womb the best possible nutrients to prepare it to host a child. If pregnancy does not occur the endometrium becomes Ama, a foreign body which the womb must expel. The body takes advantage of this to append to the menstrual flow all the filth which collected in Blood over the month. Even if a woman's digestion is not optimal in her gut she gets a second chance to nourish her higher Dhatus properly by this monthly Blood purification. This is probably one reason women live longer than men.

Unfortunately this is a blessing only as long as the menses is regular and adequate. If for some reason the menstrual flow is obstructed so that all filth is not eliminated from Blood, this virulent Ama perfuses the body and enhances the effects of other Ama. The spiritual practices which teach women to suppress their menstruation are thus highly pernicious. It is indeed said that a sign of spiritual advancement is the cessation of menses, but this should happen spontaneously once the system has become thoroughly purified. Premature deliberate cessation of menstruation is fraught with perils including the possibility for the production of dangerous blood clots.

Emotion is a significant causative factor of arthritis. When you are upset, oppressed by grief, insecurity, fear or some other powerful emotion, you cannot pay proper attention to what or when you eat. You may throw yourself into your work or your play for that emptiness of mind which comes with exhaustion, or you may turn to intoxicants to escape the oppression of your misery. You know how your appetite evaporates when you are angry or otherwise upset. Food eaten when you have no appetite creates Ama, and acts as an insidious poison whose effects surface only gradually.

Unstable emotion can cause damage by making the mind seek escape from its condition through obsessive activity. It also affects the organism directly. For example, after an emotionally charged sporting event the rheumatic factor increases in the blood of players. The disease is three times more common in individuals who were adopted as children than in those who lived with their genetic parents.

In psychotic arthritics, symptoms of arthritis alternate with symptoms of psychosis, indicating that arthritis is one means the organism has to manifest severe mental distress without totally disrupting its balance of mind. The principal result of arthritis is severe crippling which prevents the patient from living a normal life. In this it is very much like catatonia. Catatonics cannot move for psychological reasons. Arthritis sufferers have physical reasons for their immobility, and physical disability is much more socially acceptable than is mental disorder.

Arthritis sufferers are often psychologically rigid and inflexible. Suppose you are engaged in work you dislike, or you resent your boss, or you find your working conditions intolerable. If you will not adapt, and if you will not admit to yourself your inability to adapt, an attack of arthritis gives you a valid excuse to disengage yourself from work without any blame, since physical disease is supposedly "beyond your control."

Any intolerable role can result in physical stiffness which prevents or limits the necessity to play that role. Perhaps women are more prone to rheumatoid arthritis than are men, despite the fact that female sex hormones help alleviate the disease, because of Ahamkara's confusion in determining their place in life. A woman who resents having to be submissive to her husband, or who despises the dependent role her society foists on her, is pulled in two directions. Drawn by desire for both individuality and union with family and society, she is impaled on the horns of a dilemma. A physical condition helps her retain her fantasies of how she would live her life if she was free of restraint without forcing her to act on those dreams. She knows inside how she wants to be, but may lack the courage and self-confidence to hurdle the barriers to her self-expression.

Insufficient strength to resist the influences which seek to fetter her indicates weakness of Bone, the Dhatu which permits Ahamkara to project herself into the world. Weakness of Marrow, which governs the joints, makes Ahamkara fear failure every time she considers asserting herself. Fear of the consequences of self-assertion and fear of failure to self-assert combine to immobilize her, disturbing Vata and creating Astringency, which constricts her circulation and promotes congestion. Her frustration continues to increase, magnifying the Bitterness in her being and further aggravating Vata, until finally the congestion of Ama in the joint flares into inflammation, and her arthritis manifests.

The disease is an actual entity, an alien servant the patient has created out of her Ama to work for her. Now she need no longer slave away at household chores which go unappreciated by her family because she has altered her internal reality so that she need not adapt to external reality. For some sufferers rheumatoid arthritis becomes reality, security and sanity. They almost feel that they would disintegrate, that their identities would dissolve, if they relaxed, felt, wept, and returned to face external reality.

The disease is also an addiction, a crutch which makes it possible to cope. Unfortunately it is a very poisonous crutch. Ama eventually spreads to the heart, blood vessels, eyes, lungs, and nerves, resulting in anemia, swollen lymph nodes and increased heart rate. The heart complications sometimes prove fatal. Colitis, constipation, erratic blood pressure, bronchitis, kidney stones, leg cramps, and gall bladder disease can all develop as a direct result of rheumatoid arthritis. In severe cases amyloid deposition occurs. Amyloid is the debris of attacks by white blood cells on body tissues, a type of internal Ama which can cause death by clogging the kidneys.

Nowadays most sufferers from rheumatoid arthritis cannot pinpoint the day on which their disease began, because they suppress all symptoms as they arise. The pain and stiffness in their muscles and joints increase gradually over weeks or months, accompanied by unusual tiredness and a general feeling of unease. In about one out of every ten victims, however, it still develops suddenly, following the descriptions of centuries-old Ayurvedic texts, with fever, severe malaise, body ache, indigestion, thickly furred tongue and loss of ability to taste in the mouth. The principal pathology involves swelling, redness and tenderness in one or several of the large joints. Typically the inflammation moves from joint to joint, dying back in one as it springs up in another, a symptom known as "wandering pain" in Sanskrit.

In some patients emotional causes outweigh physical influences; in others, physical causes predominate. Whatever the causation, physical medicine to expel Ama from the body is essential in management of rheumatic disease because "rheum" is central to it.

Management of Arthritis

The first step in the control of rheumatoid arthritis is to acknowledge that your body is being made to undergo conflict to protect your mind from having to confront confused or repressed feelings. If you can admit to yourself that you may have such an internal conflict, and express to yourself the willingness to eventually deal with it, you can use physical therapies to control with the physical effects of the disease, confident that the hidden causes will not aggravate your condition while this physical housecleaning is going on.

You may find that this willingness to face reality is sufficient to control your disease when combined with proper physical measures, especially if your disease was mainly due to improper diet and was only secondarily due to emotional causes. Even if your emotions were the primary cause, success with your joints will increase your confidence about the possibilities for healing, making it easier to deal with your mind later when you feel ready to do so.

Like other auto-immune diseases, chronic rheumatoid arthritis displays two separate, alternating phases: exacerbation and remission. During the exacerbation phase, all the typical symptoms are present and there is acute inflammation of the joints. During remission, the symptoms disappear because the acute accumulation of the Doshas in the joints has dissipated. The Doshas are still there at the joint, threatening mayhem, but their threats are temporarily empty because they have become reduced lower than the threshold level necessary to manifest the disease. When a bucket under a tap becomes full it overflows. If you turn off the tap the bucket stops overflowing, but it is still full. As soon as the tap goes on again, even a trickle, the bucket will overflow once more.

Because there is such deep Ama in arthritic joints any Dosha accumulation in the digestive tract always tends to return to the joints and exacerbate the condition again. Health can return to the joint only after its bucket of Ama is emptied. Effective management of arthritis involves immediate elimination of Doshas during exacerbation, and gradual elimination of deep Ama during remission. The basic philosophy of therapy for rheumatoid arthritis in summarized in a pithy Sanskrit saying:

> Fasting, sweating, and the Bitter and Pungent Tastes,
> All to enkindle the digestive fire.

EXACERBATION

Fasting - Food during an exacerbation should be *light, little*, and *liquid*, in the words of Dr. Vasant Lad. Weak ginger tea sipwise, with lemon and honey if necessary, is best when your tongue is thickly coated. Proceed to rice or barley gruel, then thin mung bean soup, and finally to mung kichadi. Remain there until you go into remission, and at least a week longer, before you begin to return to your normal food. Remove all animal fats, even ghee, from your diet for two to six weeks.

You are probably allergic to several of the foods you commonly eat. After your digestion and appetite have improved, introduce only two or three new foods into your diet each day, one at each meal, and examine yourself for side-effects, like a sudden return of pain to the joint. If you are unsure about the reaction, take your pulse both before and after eating. If you pulse increases 5% or more after your meal, you are probably reacting to something that you ate. Anytime you have a reaction, eliminate that food and test it again after a week. If you still react to it, give it up for at least six months before you try it again.

Regardless of your allergies, you should eliminate all animal fats, all fried foods, all dairy products, all refrigerator cold food, all white sugar, all alcohol, and all nightshades from your diet for at least six weeks. The nightshades include potato, tomato, eggplant, peppers, and tobacco. If you cannot give tobacco up entirely, restrict yourself as much as you can. If chilies form an important part of your diet they may have caused part of the problem, and you should eliminate them during this regimen. Curtail your use of salt.

Eliminate all aluminum from your food. Aluminum is Astringent, which is why it is used in antiperspirants. It constricts body membranes and encourages Ama to dry on them, making the Ama more difficult to remove. Throw out all your aluminum cookware, and check to make sure that your baking powder is not aluminum-based.

Sweating - Because Vata is obstructed by Ama, use of ordinary oil will increase the obstruction. Castor oil alone can reduce the inflammation and scrape out the Ama. A film of castor oil should be applied on the affected joint, and then dry heat should be applied. Wet heat aggravates obstruction and congestion. A hot water bag or electric heating pad will not, but it is better to heat in the oven a tray filled with brick dust, or with a mixture of equal parts of sand and powdered rock salt, pour the heated powder into a cotton or linen bag, and apply it to the joint. The dryness of these materials helps dry out the congestion in the joint. Sunbathing is good for arthritic joints because of the healing heat of the sunrays, and because the vitamin D it creates is vital for the health of colon and Bone.

Poultices can also make the joint "sweat" by permeating it with the innate "heat" of the herbs used. Jimsonweed leaf (*Datura* species, known as stramonium or angel's trumpet in some areas) is a good, easily available material, though it is poisonous and must be used with care. The leaf can be crushed and bound over the joint with cloth, or a whole leaf can be coated with castor oil and applied after gentle roasting in a cast-iron pan. A thick paste of rhubarb root left to dry on the joint can help reduce its swelling. Paste of dry ginger helps the body digest the Ama deep in the joint. Comfrey root soothes and heals, as do slippery elm and mullein. Lobelia, pine needles, and even cayenne are all appropriate in certain circumstances. Cayenne and nettles can be used, except by Pitta people or in intense inflammation, to irritate the joint into beginning to purify itself.

Bitter and **Pungent** - These tastes are used to help control Vata and relieve Ama. In general, because Pungent is Hot in Energy it is best to use Pungent substances during remission to rekindle the digestive fire actively. Bitter substances are better during exacerbation; they rekindle digestion indirectly and help reduce inflammation. Bitter is especially needed when there is severe and generalized body ache, loss of appetite, lack of taste in the mouth, indigestion, and fever.

Fever is the body's way of sending heat to the Dhatus to help digest Ama. Even modern medicine has finally realized that fever is an important mechanism for destroying pathological microbes and viruses. Fever should be suppressed, with cold compresses, only if it climbs too high, usually above 101°F. Bitter substances catalyze fever's digestive action on Ama and permit the fever to finish work and subside sooner.

Some commonly available substances which are wholly or partly Bitter include:

Alfalfa	Chickwood	Licorice Root
Aloe Vera	Chicory	Red Clover
Bayberry	Devil's Claw	Skullcap
Birch	Echinacea	Yarrow
Burdock	Gentian	Yellow Dock
Chapparal	Golden Seal	Yucca

All Bitter substances can benefit arthritis at this stage, though each has specific properties. Gentian is useful when there is significant loss of appetite along with indigestion. Aloe Vera soothes the digestive tract and purifies the liver, as does Bayberry. Alfalfa is a natural pain reliever and purifies the colon. Devil's Claw, Yucca and Chapparal help relieve intense joint pain. Licorice Root exerts a cortisone-like effect. Skullcap soothes nerve irritation. Bayberry, Echinacea and Golden Seal help eliminate parasitic micro-organisms.

All Bitter substances help reduce the tendency to allergy by toning and rebalancing the metabolism. Ayurvedic compounds like Tikta or Mahasudarshan Churna, both of which are extremely Bitter, actively help eliminate the allergic state from your system if used regularly for at least six weeks. Such substances can also interrupt or prevent certain allergic reactions.

Guggulu is the substance of choice to control inflammation in rheumatoid arthritis. It is mainly Bitter in Taste, though its secondary Tastes are Pungent, Astringent, and Sweet. Its Energy is Hot, and its Post-Digestive Effect is Pungent. Triphala Guggulu is often useful in such conditions, since Triphala purifies the system and Trikatu improves its digestion.

The best compound of Guggulu for use in an exacerbation of rheumatoid arthritis is, however, Simhanada Guggulu. It contains Makshika Bhasma, Triphala, Sulfur, Guggulu, and castor oil, all prepared together in an iron pot. Makshika Bhasma is incinerated pyrite, which contains iron and sulfur. Iron scrapes Ama from the tissues; sulfur purifies Blood. Guggulu scrapes Ama from the joints, exerts an anti-inflammatory effect, and improves metabolism of Fat. All these substances are rejuvenators.

Castor oil is a specific for rheumatoid conditions. A Sanskrit verse states:

"The lion of castor oil alone can kill the maddened elephant of rheumatism as it stampedes through the body."

The word "Simhanada" translates as "lion's roar." Castor oil increases digestion by controlling Vata and scraping Ama from colon and Bone. If the digestive tract is coated with Ama it is wise to begin therapy by giving 2 to 4 Tbsp. of castor oil plus a cup of strong tea of dry ginger to thoroughly flush the colon and give a head start to purification of the joints.

Castor oil is Pungent, as is sulfur and, to some extent, Guggulu. Pungent items can readily be used even in an exacerbation if there is much Ama which needs to be eliminated, and if there is no intense inflammation or other symptom of great involvement of Pitta. P people, except when full of Ama, must be wary of most Pungent substances.

Common Pungent herbs include:

Angelica	Garlic	Peppermint
Calamus Root	Ginger	Spearmint
Catnip	Lobelia	Turmeric
Fennel	Mugwort	Valerian
Fenugreek	Parsley	Wood Betony

Although Pungent the mints generally do not increase Pitta unless they are used in excess. This is also the case for Turmeric.

One simple recipe for rheumatic complaints, especially those involving only one joint, is to grind a clove of Garlic in a tablespoon of milk and consume it just before bedtime. Although dairy products are specifically forbidden in this condition, this tiny amount of milk acts as a vehicle for the Garlic, and reduces its hot, irritating qualities.

In extreme inflammation, when Pitta is exceedingly increased, it is better to use Kaishora Guggulu, a form of Guggulu prepared with the herb Guduchi which reduces Guggulu's Hot and Pungent qualities.

REMISSION

Eating a balanced, anti-allergenic diet is the sort of fasting appropriate when the exacerbation diminishes. Wet heat can be used. Good Ayurvedic oils for rheumatic conditions are Dhanwantram Taila, Ksheerabala Taila, Sahachara Taila, and Vishagarbha Taila. Vishagarbha Taila, which is poisonous, is useful even during an exacerbation. All these oils are medicated to purify and lubricate the joint. Occasional medicated enemas, especially when bowel habits change and the lower tract is full of gas, are important to keep the lining of the colon healthy and clear of Ama.

Guggulu is useful during remission to remove old, adherent Ama from the Dhatus. The best varieties here are Yogaraja Guggulu and Mahayogaraja Guggulu. Both contain more than two dozen Pungent herbs for improving digestion, but Mahayogaraja also has minerals in it for a greater rejuvenating effect.

During exacerbation it is sometimes necessary to stay in bed until the joint inflammation dies down. Moving an inflamed joint too vigorously may damage it further, and may push the Ama deeper into it. Once inflammation recedes the joint must be kept mobile to minimize muscular atrophy, and to circulate the synovial fluid within it. When this circulation is interrupted, toxic Ama has an opportunity to accumulate and induce fresh inflammation.

Simple Yoga postures and breathing exercises encourage elimination of Ama. As your health improves supplement the Yoga with energetic exercise. A regular exercise program is especially important for arthritis sufferers who are overweight, since heavy limbs put extra strain on muscles and joints.

Some people notice that a pleasurable sexual experience temporarily removes arthritis pain. This happens because of a combination of psychological effect and release of endorphins in the brain. While sex may occasionally be used for quick relief, it is unwise to use sex as a painkiller habitually, because excessive sexual activity weakens the nerves and exhausts Ojas, which weakens digestion, increases Ama, and worsens the arthritis. Do not pay for short-term relief with long-term misery.

Cortisone and other anti-inflammatory drugs like phenylbutazone are other common short-terms measures which may on occasion be necessary to prevent severe joint damage. They must not be used habitually, though, because they do not address the Ama which is the cause of the condition. Drugs like cortisone are actually bribes to the immune system so that it will look the other way while more Ama is smuggled into the Dhatus. If you are using corticosteroids regularly you must *never* stop them suddenly; this can be extremely dangerous. You must taper off from them very gradually under professional supervision.

Once in remission you should deal with your emotional conflicts. Perhaps the situation existed at one time but no longer exists now. Perhaps the cause of your disease was a past experience, and your suffering is its delayed effect. If you look into yourself and find no deep confusion, it may have disappeared after creating in you the alien being which now ravages you.

If you do locate an emotional maelstrom you must examine it without prejudice. The Bitter Taste in your supplements will help you admit your dissatisfaction to yourself. There is no benefit in assigning blame for that dissatisfaction. Dealing with present reality by determining your current needs and considering how to obtain them is more important. If you are having difficulty being objective about your situation, ask for help from a trusted friend or a professional counselor. Do not make a habit of emotional purgation lest it begin to intensify your misery, just as overuse of the Pungent Taste increases Pitta and therefore anger.

Do not empower the alien personality you have created for yourself by giving it more importance than it is worth. You created it to do a job for you, and it did its job. Now that you have no further need of it you can allow it to go. As Ama departs and the Dhatus return to health Ahamkara will become stronger and you will be able to find in your "self" the satisfaction you may not have been able to locate externally. Love and compassion for yourself are the strongest remedies which exist for any disease, and the best nourishment for your immune system.

Cancer

Love and compassion are even more important in malignancy. As in rheumatoid arthritis, an alien personality is created. In arthritis the entity, like a good slave, performs the function it was created for. In cancer the alien alterego rebels and turns on its maker. Taking over a renegade cell, the rebel proliferates, creates a body for itself, and challenges Ahamkara in a cancerous civil war for possession of the organism. If Ahamkara gives in and admits that all is lost, the cancer becomes terminal.

It seems amazing that Ahamkara, who adores life and tries to stay alive as long as she possibly can, could surrender and relinquish her authority to a murderous upstart. Sometimes overwhelming physical pollution which makes the body uninhabitable, such as intense or long-term exposure to chemical carcinogens or to radiation, is the cause. Sometimes an individual whose digestion has been impaired for many years develops cancer because of ancient residual Ama. And sometimes extreme hopelessness can so overwhelm Ahamkara and the immune system that a cancer arises.

The power of hopelessness is such that even people who have well-integrated personalities may develop cancers if the shock of some loss is too intense. Even a temporary spell of hopelessness may be sufficient to initiate a cancerous chain of events in someone whose body is filled with life-long physical Ama accumulation. And, exposure to powerful chemical or radioactive carcinogens engender hopelessness in the cells of the body, who sense the fatal implications of the exposure. This cellular hopelessness is eventually fatal to the personality.

The health of Blood, which provides invigoration to Ahamkara, is critical to cancer development. In fact hemolysis, or destruction of the blood, is common in cancer. Ayurveda draws a distinction between "red" and "white" Blood. As long as Blood is full of healthy red cells it nourishes and invigorates all the Dhatus and provides them Prana.

When Blood becomes filled with the white cells of the immune system, which shows that the system has shifted its emphasis from nutrition of the Dhatus to elimination of Ama and aliens, it cannot provide proper invigoration. Lack of Prana, transported by oxygen, encourages the growth of cancerous tissue, which hates oxygen. "White Blood" encourages hopelessness at the cellular level.

A cancer usually results when an individual undergoes a physical or mental experience which is utterly indigestible by the personality, something which the being cannot face under any circumstances. That forever alien experience lies in wait in the organism until it finds an abnormal, rebellious cell in which to live, and an invader is born. By being so unwilling to face reality, Ahamkara herself isolates and provides identity and individuality to this indigestible fact.

When this "individual" finds a suitable host cell it "possesses" it, as a disembodied spirit might possess a human being. Because the fact is unbearable to Ahamkara it is categorized as disruptive or "evil" from the onset, so when it is let loose in the body it destroys, true to the role assigned it. Cancer is too often a self-fulfilling prophecy. Even the belief that "everyone else can get cancer, but not me," a sign of mental indigestion, often masks a strong subconscious fear of that very event.

Cancer production usually involves many factors in varying degrees of influence. Common to all cancers, however, is the incubation of initiating substances (carcinogens) in damaged cells and the possession of these cells by a self-generated alien personality. Sometimes Ama itself can act as a carcinogen. Even if it does not, Ama is essential for cancer proliferation because it is undigested material. Undigested thought and undigested food naturally gravitate to one another and nourish one another. Cancer cells receive their physical nourishment from Ama irrigation and their mental encouragement from hopelessness.

It has been reported that a majority of cancer patients were not breast-fed. This may deprive them of some essential immune substance carried in the breast milk, or it may deprive them of early bonding with their mothers, or both. Good bonding with others begins with a good maternal bond. Poor bonding with others usually affects Ahamkara's ability to bind to the Dhatus, and encourages alien cells to bind instead.

A potential cancer patient may feel early on a deep sense of existential loneliness in his or her life, and may erect barriers to keep others from loving them. They may give much more than they receive, and may feel uncomfortable about accepting anything from others. This Astringent constriction which inhibits Salty enjoyment causes inability to accept Sweet nourishment from others, and guarantees disappointment in relationships because the giving is so needy. The Bitterness of disappointment may create unfocused Pungent anger or Sour envy. When all Tastes are sufficiently imbalanced Ahamkara may decide that life is no longer worth living.

Some people use a gun, a noose or pills to commit suicide when the last straw drops onto them; others commit psychic suicide, and withdraw from the world into schizophrenia. Some cancer-prone people invite a malignant hit man into them to legitimize their longing for sympathy from others. They allow themselves to accept assistance because of the disease, which is supposedly not their fault.

Any powerful dissatisfaction can affect Ahamkara. Cervical cancer strikes most often either women who are lifelong virgins, or those who are extremely sexually promiscuous. The former shun a pleasure which they feel they do not deserve, the latter embrace the pleasure but ensure that they do not receive real fulfillment from it, which they are sure they do not deserve. Men who suffer from such sexual uncertainty are likewise more prone to prostate cancer.

Such emotionally cancer-prone individuals often find some reason for living outside themselves. It may be an individual, like a spouse, or some situation, like a job. They then become addicted to it, investing everything they have in that external crutch, empowering it totally. Loss of this investment is a crushing blow, because Ahamkara has to quit her addiction cold turkey. Unless some substitute can be found terminal despair and final dejection may set in, and the stage is set for one of the 100,000 cancer cells which arise each day in the body to establish its own regime.

These cells may begin in any Dhatu, though when a cancer is unchecked it eventually eats through them all. Vata makes cancer cells abnormal, and makes them proliferate rapidly. Kapha provides the uncontrolled increase in cell mass, and Pitta is in charge of robbing nutrition from other Dhatus to feed the interloper. Cancer is at once a tornado of Vata which disrupts normal bodily functions and structures, a raging forest fire of Pitta which consumes the Dhatus, and a great tidal wave of Kapha whose flood inundates all Dhatus with its Ama-poison. The Doshas, which preserve the body in peaceful times, destroy it when disease gains control of them.

Consumption

This disease category represents several terminal conditions, among them tuberculosis and AIDS. It is also called "emaciation," or "chronic wasting syndrome," descriptions which are regarded as diagnostic of AIDS infection in a virus carrier. Ayurveda calls it consumption because it occurs when a disease completely overruns an individual, "consuming" him or her. As in cancer, all Doshas, all Dhatus and all Tastes are disturbed in this condition, which differs from cancer in that a consumptive's mindset is the precise opposite of a cancer patient's. Consumptives and cancer patients both have loneliness in common, but consumptives never doubt their self-worth. They are sure that they deserve the enjoyments of life, and put their wishes and desires before those of anyone else. They take what they want, regardless of the result.

The chief cause of consumption is willfulness. Consumptive types think they can do anything, and terminally overstrain themselves in order to prove it. Here Ahamkara is so overconcerned with sensory gratification that she indulges in repeated "crimes against wisdom" and neglects to properly nourish her body.

Consumption develops in one of two ways. Taking in more nutrients of any sort than you can digest, particularly by excessive indulgence in improper diet, fills the system up with Ama and aggravates Kapha. Excessive indulgence in exercise or sex, excessive discipline like fanatic fasting and penance, or excessive use of tobacco, alcohol, drugs, and other intoxicants exhaust Ojas, starve the Dhatus and aggravate Vata. Continual restraint of any natural urge also disturbs Vata. The thirteen natural urges which must never be restrained are the urges to: urinate, defecate, fart, vomit, sneeze, belch, yawn, ejaculate semen when aroused, eat when hungry, drink when thirsty, sleep when tired, pant when exhausted, and cry when miserable.

Common to all these causes is "too much." Ahamkara tries too hard to show off, to demonstrate that she is better, brighter, stronger, smarter, tougher, more talented, and generally more valuable than anyone else in the world. She tries to exceed herself, but succeeds only in exceeding her limitations.

Excessive nutrition causes Kapha and Ama to block the pathways for Dhatu nutrition, and obstructs the proper movement of nutrients, which is controlled by Vata. Insufficient intake of nutrients to replace an excessive outflow of energy, especially from repetitive, unsatisfying sex, directly disturbs Vata, whose dry, light and rough qualities exhaust the Dhatus. Both processes rob the Dhatus of nourishment, decrease Ojas, and weaken the immunity, permitting parasitical beings to colonize the system. The problem is not tubercle bacilli, Candida yeast, the Epstein-Barr virus, or even the AIDS virus. The problem is immune weakness, which is due to aggravated Vata.

We Americans guard our commitment to excess as if to prove our individuality to ourselves. Our gas guzzlers must be bigger than anyone else's; our GNP must be most colossal. We enjoy and enjoy, with no thought for tomorrow or for anyone else's tomorrow. We organize our lives around bread and circuses. But we cannot forever expand our indulgences, any more than we can endlessly expand our economy, because the disease of consumption lies in wait for all who overconsume and attempt to aggrandize themselves at the expense of the rest of Nature's creation.

There is no single therapy for cancer and consumption. The Ayurvedic approach to both involves whittling away at the strength of the disease while rebuilding the individual's immune power, to create a climate in which Nature can cure. Whatever the therapy, rejuvenation is essential to invigorate the Dhatus and revitalize the organism.

In potentially fatal diseases like cancer and consumption the normal sequence of treatment steps is reversed. When you are injured in an accident you must initially get first aid for the injury, and then worry about everything else. Likewise, in serious disease you may first have to preserve life and only then consider how to purify and balance the system.

Therefore, for cancer and consumption, our procedure often becomes:

Rejuvenation first:
to preserve life.

Balancing the Doshas second:
to strengthen the patient and weaken the disease.

Panchakarma next:
to purify the system.

Removal of the emotional cause of the condition thereafter:
when the patient is ready for it.

This may hold true even if the disease is not yet grave, especially when a mental predisposition is the main cause. One of my friends complained that when the pressure to "achieve"—in her work, in her relationship— mounted in her it would eventually create a fever. The fever would burn away all her accumulated nervous energy and leave her temporarily relaxed, but would return again and again. She asked my advice.

I told her that a major portion of her difficulty was due to her insistence on trying to use her will force to solve her problems. When her boss complained or her boyfriend argued she would throw herself into the situation in an assault on the walls preventing free communication.

After reminding her that the only result you can expect from beating your head on a brick wall is a sore skull, I suggested that she first *rejuvenate* herself, with nourishing herbs and with her favorite activities, and put all else on hold when she felt the fever rising. Once the crisis passed, I suggested that she *balance* the energy of interaction with the boss or the boyfriend, and once calm had returned that only then should she try to *purify* the relationship by *removing the cause* of the disagreement.

If you fail to relax and regroup when stress hits you, your imbalances will age you quickly; stress will *consume* you. Systematic rejuvenation is the best answer for the problem of the unnatural stresses of our modern lives.

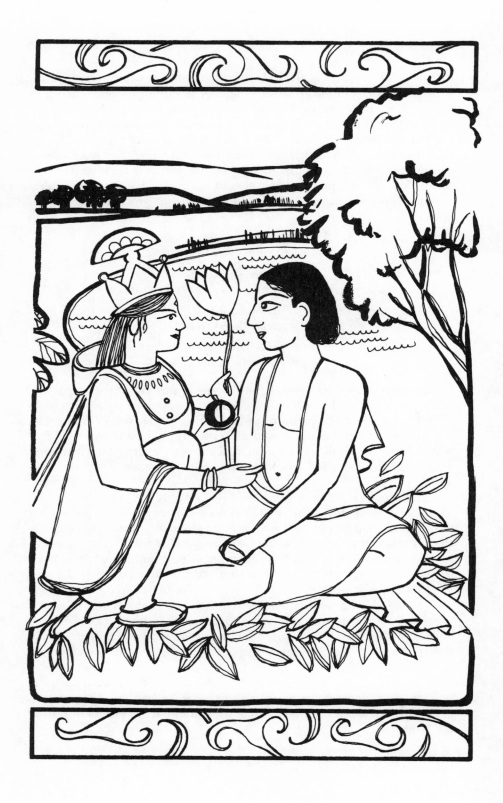

Chapter Eight

Rejuvenation

Disease always forces us to confront our attachments. All attachments are temporary, and are dissolved by Nature when She feels it is time to broaden our personalities. Disease is always an opportunity to learn from our mistakes, an opportunity given by Nature out of Her maternal magnanimity. She hopes we will learn enough that we need never be sick. She can even teach us how to overcome death, and to develop permanent personalities like the immortals. Rejuvenation is the first step in the direction of immortality.

Old age is an auto-immune disease, an admission by Ahamkara that she is no longer adequately able to identify with the body. Old age is caused by repeated indulgence in sensory pleasures, whose wear and tear on the body destroys Ojas. The faster your life, the faster you deteriorate. A hummingbird flits just a few seasons; a tortoise plods along for decades. Longevity requires slowness. When your life is slow your protective aura can interpose itself efficiently between you and the outside world.

The word for rejuvenation in Ayurveda is Rasayana, which literally means "the Path of Rasa." To walk the Path of Rasa you must purify and nourish your physical Rasa Dhatu, since Rasa is the raw material from which the other Dhatus are formed. Healthy Rasa Dhatu is the first step in the physical production of healthy Shukra, from which Ojas is directly produced. Careful selection of food tastes (Rasas) and control of emotions (Rasas) ensures production of healthy Rasa Dhatu, and therefore healthy Shukra and Ojas.

Because Shukra is best nourished by Sweet, rejuvenation requires creation of powerful Sweetness in body and mind. Honey is made of pollen, the sperm of plants. Plant Shukra increases human Shukra, according to the principle "like increases like." Honey is, therefore, innately rejuvenating. In addition, honey is a predigested food, thanks to those industrious bees, and it can enter any part of the body without having to be first digested. It can do this for any medicine mixed with it, which is why it is valued as the best of all vehicles for therapeutic and rejuvenating substances.

Mixing raw, unfiltered honey into your herbal tea allows honey to act as a vehicle for the active principles of the herb. Because honey is made poisonous by heating, however, it should be added after the tea is brewed and has cooled to the temperature at which you will drink it. In honor of its position as the ideal Sweet food, honey is called "Madhu" in Sanskrit. "Madhu" means perfection of Sweet, in contrast to "Madhura," which refers to Sweet which must be first digested before it can give its Sweetness to Ahamkara. All other physical substances are merely Madhura; only honey is Madhu.

Virilization

Most rejuvenators including honey are also aphrodisiacs, because both classes of substances increase Shukra Dhatu. A tremendous increase in Shukra usually inflames the fires of lust and causes a craving for sexual gratification. If you want a rejuvenating effect you must avoid arousal and contain the energy within you so that it can be digested into Ojas.

Onions increase Shukra quickly. But because they promote Rajas, or mental activity, they make it much more difficult to contain the Shukra long enough to convert it into Ojas. Onions produce Shukra, but also cause the mind to search for a sexual situation in which to expend it. Ghee, the metal gold, and mercury sulfide also produce Shukra quickly, and also increase Rajas, though they and honey are less Rajas-producing than are onions.

Ayurveda separates the sciences of virilization and rejuvenation because virilization, besides increasing Shukra, also involves techniques for enhancing both sexual pleasure and fertility. Mutual pleasure is essential in sex; in fact, Charak, the chief Ayurvedic author, says that the best of all virilizers is a partner who loves you. Sex is more important to a woman than it is to a man, say the ancient texts. Modern medicine has in fact found that male pheromones, imbibed by a woman during the sex act, help regulate her fertility and ensure the health of her reproductive system. Regular sexual intercourse improves a woman's well-being.

Unsatisfactory sex is the cause of much disease in today's world, especially among women. A woman has every right to become angry if her man fails to satisfy her sexually, because he is withholding essential nutrients from her. Inadequate nutrition increases Vata, making her periods more erratic and difficult. Sexual frustration creates anger, and the Pungency created by anger imbalances a female's sexual organs and Blood and further affects her menstruation. Menstrual disturbances heighten a woman's emotional aggravation.

It is difficult for such a woman to become pregnant, and should she become pregnant her misery will be transferred to the child in her womb by the toxins circulating in her impure blood. Any baby grown in such a Bitter and Pungent environment will grow up dissatisfied and angry because those emotions are the foundation of that child's constitution.

Virilization is rejuvenation for Shukra Dhatu, and it is "pre-juvenation" for your children. Virilization is a method for selecting the healthiest possible genes a couple can muster to create a child with the healthiest possible constitution. This art of loving strengthens the male and female bodies and creates in them maximum excitement at the moment of congress. Some of that joy and excitement is transmitted into the zygote and provides a foundation of satisfaction on which the child can base its life.

Desire is the first disease, says the Ayurvedic writer Vagbhata. If a zygote can be infused with some of the immense satisfaction that a couple feels at the moment of orgasm, the child who develops will be more easily satisfied with life than the child whose parents were convulsed by powerful, twisted emotions at the time of conception, leaving it with constitutional hungers it can never satiate.

The foundation of sexual stress is loss of Ojas, which is itself caused by sexual overindulgence. Many modern couples fail to take the time to properly enjoy sex, and seek only self-gratification instead of mutual satisfaction. Masturbation is the culmination of this tendency, the apex of self-indulgence and gratuitous waste of energy. The repetitious performance of unsatisfying sex is certain to cause disease.

Individuals lose the willingness to surrender themselves to each other in sexual union when they feel vulnerable because of weak identities. Lack of Ojas, due especially to frequent obsessive sex, weakens the aura, and whenever anyone gets too close subliminal alarm bells begin to go off. Every personality is organized differently, and the melding of auras which occurs when two people unite sexually is inherently threatening to Ahamkara. If she has been weakened by weak Ojas she feels overwhelmed by the opposing personality, sensing that her defenses are insufficient to protect herself, and may paroxysmally thrust the partner away, physically or emotionally.

Many degrees of rejuvenation exist, but rejuvenation even to a minor degree is possible only when you discipline your sexual activity. Since sex is the third Pillar of Life your attitude to sex must reflect its importance to your health. Reverence for sex is the real significance behind the philosophy of sexual restraint called Brahmacharya, which literally means "that which brings you closer to the Creator." Yogis interpret this in a religious sense and follow the path of celibacy. Ayurveda interprets it to mean "that which causes the Creative Energy of the universe to accumulate within you."

Sex is the Pillar of Life most closely associated with Vata. Orgasmic sex is a tremendous energy drain on the system. Castrated salmon, for example, live twice as long as their potent counterparts simply because they do not exhaust themselves sexually. Sexual activity must always be carefully regulated lest it vitiate Vata.

It is best, for example, to enjoy sex at night, since night is ruled by

Kapha, and Vata disturbance is less likely to result from sexual exertion then. Ayurveda suggests that orgasmic sex be limited to not more than twice a week in winter, when the body's internal fire is highest. In the spring and fall once a week is the suggested maximum frequency, and in summer, when the body is ravaged by heat, sex is indicated only once every two weeks. Yogis are even stricter, suggesting no more than once a month. Everyone should abstain from sex during illness and convalescence, and during menstruation.

Because the frequency of sexual activity should be limited to preserve physical health, and because unsatisfactory sex is an important cause of disease, the quality of each sexual experience must be enhanced. Meditation alone can do this. Sex itself should be made into a meditation, or an act of ritual worship, which can actually increase Ojas instead of decreasing it.

One of the Upanishads, spiritual treatises which explain the hidden meanings of the Vedas, describes all life in the cosmos in terms of sacrifice into fire. The world beyond is a form of the universal Fire, as is our world, and the gods send rain to transmit water from the one to the other. In the internal cosmos of the human body, the world beyond is the brain, the rain is the Ojas, and the gods are the mind and the senses. Our world is the physical body.

A human body is also a fire. Its open mouth is the fuel, its breath the smoke, its speech the flame, its eyes the coals, its ears the sparks. Into this fire, which represents the digestive processes in the Dhatus, the gods offer food; from this offering arises Shukra. A woman's body has a special fire, a sexual fire. During intercourse the penis is the fuel, the pubic hairs the smoke, the vulva the flame, penetration the coals, and pleasure the sparks. Into this fire the gods offer semen. From this offering arises a new human being.

Two people performing sex should sacrifice all restraint, all doubts and uncertainties which separate them from each other and prevent them from becoming one, into the momentary unity experience of orgasm. Until you can convert your sexual experiences into meditations you will always be tempted to search for new sexual partners to satisfy your appetites, never able to locate that total sense of satisfaction which ordinary sex hints at but cannot achieve.

Successful sexual satisfaction occurs between two partners, not between two genital organs. It does not happen immediately, but grows and develops over time. The first step in improving your sexual experience is to resist the temptation to hop from bed to bed to seek improved pleasure. You must stick to one partner. V people are tempted by variety more than are other types; they should satisfy this craving for variation with new techniques and positions, not with new partners.

P people also have roving eyes, but their principal urge is for intensity of experience, and not variation. They have to be careful not to completely dominate a weaker partner, or worse, to permit their craving for intensity to mesmerize them into perversion. K people are least likely to roam, and since sex is a good vigorous exercise for them they can be encouraged to enjoy it more often than Ps or Vs, for whom ordinary sex is more a luxury than it is for Ks.

The first step in any virilization program must be absolute sexual chastity for a month or more. It takes at least a month for the body to rebuild its Ojas stores so that Ahamkara can feel sufficiently secure within herself to permit another being to come into intimate contact with her. Selective chastity, the practice of observing physical continence while actively fantasizing about sex, is useless. Sex is all in the brain anyway; no excitement occurs unless the mind wills it to occur. The continuous pressure of unresolved sexual thoughts is more detrimental to Ojas than is the physical loss of Ojas during the sex act. Moreover, the mental duplicity and deception involved leads to deviousness, which promotes willfulness and encourages other diseases to develop.

As with rejuvenation, full purification must precede virilization. Thereafter medicated oils should be applied regularly to the genitals to nourish and invigorate them. Internally, dates, nutmeg, clove, gold, Pippali (long pepper), Shatavari (asparagus root), and licorice root are among the substances used in virilizing recipes. When two people come together to unite themselves sexually, they should prepare for themselves a well-appointed bedchamber with Sweet music, Sweet fragrances, and Sweet flowers to look at, to nourish and satisfy the mind and all the senses. Flowers are the sex organs of plants, and their presence enhances the effect.

The full moon night is the best of all nights for sexual union, if the woman is not menstruating, because the moon floods the mind with Rasa. Lunar eclipses and new moon nights, on which the natural lunar luminescence is darkened, are meant for meditation, not sexual excitement. Every other night of the month is permissible, and each night the experience will differ, according to the phase of the moon. Whichever night is chosen, the couple should don clean, Sweet-smelling clothes after a good bath, and should then eat a light meal of Sweet foods, with a little wine. Because sex, like exercise, should not be performed immediately after eating, the couple should engage themselves in dalliance for an hour or more before becoming truly passionate.

All this Sweetness, coupled with a gay, carefree attitude, ensures a wonderful experience, and, if conception should occur, a wonderful child. The ancient texts describe 84 positions for sexual pleasure. If conception is desired, male-on-top positions are best, because they allow the sperm to reach the ovum with least obstruction, and make it easier for the zygote to implant itself in the wall of the womb. Whether or not conception is the object of the union, the male must maintain firm control of himself so that his partner can satiate herself with pleasure.

After sex, you should urinate, to expel any residual Vata from your pelvis, and take a hot bath, to relax your body. It is good to do one or two Yoga asanas to balance Vata. Both partners should then drink a cup of hot milk with dates, slivered almonds, ghee, honey, and saffron, to replenish the Shukra which has been expended. Milk, ghee, and honey all enhance Ojas, but milk is the best of all substances to nourish Shukra quickly. Be sure not to use ghee and honey in equal amounts. If one or both partners are allergic to milk almond milk can be used instead.

Rasayana

Increase in Shukra is also the goal of physical rejuvenation, which requires strict discipline. The effect you obtain is directly proportional to the discipline you follow. Some self-controlled people use discipline alone for rejuvenation, and utilize their inherent Prana, Tejas and Ojas for transmutation. Modern research has proven that there are two guaranteed ways to live longer: decrease your body temperature, and decrease your food intake. It has been estimated that if normal body temperature could be reduced by a mere 3°F we could live an extra 30 years. More years can be added by reducing your food intake to the minimum required for good nutrition. Vitamins and minerals can help you only indirectly. Aerobics can strengthen your body and increase its stamina, but it cannot increase your lifespan.

When Yogis sit in meditation for years in the intense cold of the High Himalaya, ingesting as little as possible, their Yoga and their passive acceptance of the external cold cools their bodies and preserves them far longer than they could preserve themselves in a polluted, stress-filled environment like a city. Their aims also differ from ours: they seek longer life to permit them to perfect their meditations.

This is why Yogis worship the great Lord Shiva. Shiva is not a god in the normal sense of the English word; He is the personification of the power of transformation. Shiva has the power to transform anything He likes. He is called the God of Death because His transformations are so intense that most beings who undergo them are unable to maintain their Ahamkara-integrity and must dissolve instead.

Shiva is always portrayed as a Yogi on Mt. Kailas, the holiest of all pilgrimage spots for Hindus and Buddhists alike. Like all the High Himalayas, Mt. Kailas is intensely cold. Heat causes dilation of all sensory channels, to permit the organism to project its mind into the external world and experience its sense objects. Cold constricts these sensory channels and impedes this projection of mind. When Ahamkara is filled with desire for experience, she heats up the mind and body to prepare them for sensory experiences. As desire dies, mind and body cool and the senses turn inward.

Ordinary exposure to cold or cold emotions like fear strips fire from the body because its heat is diffused throughout all its tissues. Yogis practice Yoga for decades to gradually constrict all their channels evenly and smoothly, which concentrates their fire deep within where it is safe from all external influences. Simultaneously they perfect their internal concentration sufficiently to withstand the power of Shiva's transformation. Anyone interested in rejuvenation must learn internal concentration, which my teacher Vimalananda referred to as "interiority."

All mental and physical strain must be eliminated from your life if you hope to rejuvenate yourself through discipline alone. You must cultivate internal and external calm and quiet in a stabilized mind with a firm mental disposition. Some Yogis follow these restrictions alone in their caves in the towering mountains. If you cannot control your emotions perfectly, you will be unable to rejuvenate yourself with discipline alone, because fiery emotion will burn away your Ojas as it collects, and frigid emotion will dry it up.

Strict dietary control is essential. Hot Tastes, which direct the consciousness externally, must be eliminated from the diet. Alcohol and all other intoxicants, all Pungent, Sour and Salty food and drink, and anger, hatred and all other such divisive emotions must be avoided. Astringency and its accompanying fear must be eliminated to keep the channels of nutrition unconstricted. Even Bitter, which is essential for bringing the Doshas into balance, must be removed from this diet. Only Sweet is permitted. Fresh cow's milk, cow's ghee, and honey are the three most important rejuvenating foods for use in a discipline-oriented rejuvenation program.

Perfect physical and mental discipline is one way of withdrawing from the world. You simply refuse to allow provocation to affect you. If you still fall prey to emotional upset occasionally you will have to physically retreat from the world for some time to avoid provocations which might agitate your mind and burn your Ojas. If you cannot retreat from the world forever you should try to arrange to retreat for at least a month, and you should use a rejuvenating substance to enhance the effect of your discipline. V and P types usually need substances, Vs because their dryness exhausts Ojas, and Ps because their inner fire burns Ojas. One month is really a minimum to obtain any kind of significant effect, although any retreat, even for a day, is bound to be beneficial.

Ideally, you should avoid all human contact during your retreat, remaining in your room, avoiding even wind and sun. Isolation from the external world helps you balance your internal existence. Thorough Panchakarma purification is needed before you begin, and careful regulation of your food and sleep is essential. Sex is banned during the rejuvenation period. This may sound boring, but rejuvenation cannot occur in an atmosphere of perpetual stimulation and excitement. You cannot be "busy" rejuvenating any more than a tree can be busy growing. Rejuvenation, like growth, happens at Nature's pace.

A rejuvenating substance can enhance the effects of your discipline even if you are unable to go on retreat. It should be consumed early in the morning well before breakfast so that it need not compete with food for digestion, and so that any abnormal metabolism or emotions which might develop during the day will not disturb the rejuvenating effect. You must consume the substance for at least three weeks for it to have a minimal effect; six weeks is even better. During this period you must avoid everything you would avoid during convalescence, including extensive travel, loud or extensive speaking, violent behavior, and any other Vata-disturbing activities that would destroy Ojas. Meditation and mild exercise are desirable.

Some simple rejuvenating formulas:

Crush seven *black peppercorns* and mix their powder with honey. Yogis like black pepper because its drying effect dries reproductive secretions and helps preserve celibacy. It also dries other body secretions, and is a good rejuvenator for those who have weak lungs which are easily clogged by Kapha. This is better for K, VK, and PK types than it is for Vs, VPs and Ps.

Pippali, or *long pepper*, is a specific rejuvenator for the lungs. Although it is Pungent in Taste and Hot in Energy, it is Sweet in Post-Digestive Effect. Because it is oily it can increase Kapha if used continuously for several months. Misuse of Pippali can increase all Three Doshas.

Soak one handful of *chickpeas* overnight in water and slowly chew and swallow them the next morning, washing them down with the soak water. This is especially good for weakness of the stomach.

Gently heat 1 tsp. of *powdered licorice root* in 1 cup milk; do not boil. Drink twice daily. Avoid long-term use of licorice root if you have high blood pressure. Licorice root is especially good for the sexual organs.

Shatavari, a variety of *asparagus root*, is especially rejuvenative for the female reproductive organs. 1 tsp. simmered 5 to 10 minutes in a cup of milk with 1/4 tsp. powdered ginger and a finely chopped Medjool date is good for both V and P types.

Garlic is rejuvenating for V and K types especially. It has five Tastes— all except Sour—but Pungent and Sweet predominate. It is Hot in Energy and Pungent in Post-Digestive Effect. Green garlic, which is plucked after only a couple of weeks of life when it has its first long green leaves and is used as the whole plant, is much milder, far less likely to aggravate Pitta, and much less disturbing to the mind than is ordinary garlic. You must always reduce dry garlic's intensity by sauteing it for 30 seconds in ghee or unsalted butter. P and V types can also simmer it 5 to 10 minutes in 1 cup milk mixed with 1/2 cup water, strain and drink.

Tulsi, or *holy basil*, is said to possess an unusually strong form of Prana within it which can treat almost any disease, including cancer. It is ideal for fevers. For prevention of Dosha imbalance 1 oz. of the juice of the fresh leaves can be taken by V and K types each morning.

Pomegranate juice is carefully evaporated into a thick syrup over a low fire. Daily 1 silver leaf and 1 gold leaf should be added to 2 tsp. of this syrup and the mixture made into a ball. This is then consumed with fresh milk, especially by individuals of advanced age, in whom retarding the ageing process is a more realistic goal than reversing it.

Gotu kola helps rejuvenate the mind and improve the memory. It is mainly Bitter in Taste, with Astringent and Sweet aftertastes, Cold in Energy, and Sweet in Post-Digestive Effect. Overuse of gotu kola can increase Vata. Gotu kola is best for V types and P types if its tea is simmered gently with ghee until all the water disappears, so that its active principles remain in the ghee, which antidotes any side-effects. K types should take it as a tea.

Triphala paste can be applied to the bottom of a clean new cast iron pan, to permit it to absorb some of the iron. After at least 24 hours it should be removed 1 tsp. at a time and consumed as a paste with honey, followed by a glass of warm water in which 1 tsp. of honey has been dissolved. This is especially good for those who need to eliminate large quantities of Ama which have accumulated over many years.

Haritaki is sometimes used alone or in preparations like Agastya Rasayana to scrape away Ama and rejuvenate simultaneously. Haritaki can cause Vata increase if used continuously for too long. It should not be given to emaciated, dried-out individuals, pregnant women, or to people who have a Pitta imbalance or who have recently hemorrhaged. It should be given with raw sugar during summer or in a hot climate, and with dry ginger or long pepper during winter or in a cold climate. In autumn, it should be mixed with rock salt, and in spring, with honey.

Fresh Amalaki fruit is most often made into jam or preserves. Amalaki Rasayana and Dhatri Rasayana are two common preparations. The most famous of all Amalaki-based rejuvenators is Chyavanprash

Avaleha. Amalaki is its main ingredient, and more than two dozen other herbs are added for synergistic effects. A sweetener, such as raw sugar, jaggery (solidified sugar cane juice), or honey, is added to provide intense, concentrated Sweet. Amalaki and the other herbs insure that the Sweet is properly digested and causes no reaction.

The dose of Chyvanprash is 1 to 2 Tbsp. each morning, followed by a cup of warm milk with saffron. Saffron must always be added after removing the milk from the fire, to preserve its potency. The best way to consume Chyvanprash is to obtain dried dates from an Indian grocery store. Soak two of these dried dates overnight. The next morning slit open the swollen dates and fill them with Chyvanprash and a blanched almond. Chew slowly.

Minerals and Metals

Minerals have been used in Ayurveda ever since Tantra began its researches into alchemy. Every mineral, like every herb, has its own Taste-personality. Gold, for example, is Sweet, silver is Sour, copper is Pungent, and iron is Astringent. Gold is the best medicine for Vata because it is Hot as well as Sweet. Silver is a good medicine for Pitta because like Amalaki it is Cold as well as Sour; its Sourness increases the digestion, while the Cold prevents Pitta from increasing. Copper controls Kapha because it is Hot as well as Pungent, and scrapes Ama and Kapha from the body. Iron nourishes Blood, and its Astringency prevents Blood from becoming too Hot or too fluid.

Gold is solidified sunrays. Its effects are like the effects of the sun. Wearing it purifies all energy entering the body. It improves the skin, the body's overall beauty, the joints, and the being's overall energy. It is a general antidote for all types of poison, including Ama. The gold salts used in modern medicine for arthritis also control Vata and help eliminate Ama from the system, but cause side-effects because they are soluble. They dissolve into reactive ions which are too intense to be safely utilized by the system.

Ayurvedic metals and minerals, including gold, are prepared in a very different way. First they are thoroughly purified, to remove any poisonous pollutants. Then pastes of medicinal herbs are applied to them and they are incinerated. Some scientists believe that the herbs form chelates with the minerals; others have different theories. What is certain is that after the incineration most of these minerals, except gold and probably silver, become oxides or sulfides.

Most metal oxides and sulfides are quite insoluble in water and so do not break up into reactive ions when they enter the body. They remain as unreactive substances within the body and seem to exert a catalytic effect on metabolic processes. Gold, and silver to a great extent, apparently remain unreacted, but the incineration reduces them into finely divided unreactive particles which act like the oxides. The main reason that other metals are converted into oxides or sulfides is to eliminate their reactivity; gold, which is practically non-reactive anyway, needs only to be divided into tiny particles.

More incinerations means smaller particle size. When the particles become sufficiently small, at least small enough to fill the lines on the fingertips, they can circulate in the system and exert their effects much longer than can ordinary medicines. This is one of the reasons minerals are useful for rejuvenation therapy. Another reason: Bhasmas (incinerated metals and minerals) become more potent with age as their particles naturally become smaller and smaller, whereas herbs lose their potency after a year or two. 100-year-old Bhasmas are highly prized in India.

The dose of a Bhasma is commonly a small heap of powder the size of a grain of rice. The intense Taste of the Bhasma is therefore not so unpleasant as is that of the larger doses needed for herbal medicine. Bhasmas also act more quickly and their effects last longer than herbs. A Bhasma is made into a paste with honey, butter, or ghee, and the paste is then put under the tongue for quicker results. The first effect of the Bhasma comes from the transmission of its Taste into the brain; the second effect, which happens almost as quickly as the first, involves the release of Prana into the bloodstream, carried by a subtle, potentiated form of oxygen created during the process of incineration. The third effect is due to the mineral itself and occurs as the particles of the Bhasma circulate throughout the body.

Traditionally, each physician prepared his or her own medicines, but with cultural modernization many physicians have elected to rely on Ayurvedic pharmaceutical manufacturers to provide them with medicines. As Ayurvedic medicines become more and more available in America, and people become tempted to try mineral preparations for rejuvenation, the question of quality becomes more and more acute. "Know your dealer" is an important watchword for those who would purchase Ayurvedic medicines. Many Ayurvedic pharmacies produce Bhasmas nowadays; not all of them produce them correctly.

For example, mica (called Abhraka in Sanskrit) Bhasma is an excellent rejuvenator for the lungs and for Rasa Dhatu. To make the best mica Bhasma you must dig a hole in the ground three feet cubical, and lay aside a store of 1500 cakes of dried cow dung. Cow dung cakes are used widely in India as fuel and to cremate corpses because they burn slowly with intense heat. After filling the pit with about 500 cakes you add a sealed clay vessel containing the mica and its herbal helpers, and then finish filling the pit with the other 1000 cakes. It will take at least a day, and usually longer, for the pile to burn itself out. After it cools the clay vessel is retrieved and opened, and the mica is prepared with herbs for its next incineration. All told, it takes about 3 days to do one incineration properly and prepare for the next.

Most minerals only require 5, 7, or 11 incinerations to prepare them for use. Mica is most powerful when it has been incinerated 100, or even 1000 times. Yogis who had unlimited time, herbs and cow dung could afford to invest the eight or more years it takes to incinerate mica properly 1000 times. Modern companies cannot, and it is better today, therefore, to use mica which has been incinerated just enough to lose all its sparkle, even though a larger dose will be necessary to do the job.

Likewise, many companies tout their diamond Bhasma as a panacea for all ills including cancer, but few people know how to make diamond Bhasma properly. Unless you can tell the difference you are as likely to be cheated over diamond Bhasma as you are over gem-quality diamonds. For this reason substitutes have been identified. If you are unable to obtain reliable diamond Bhasma you can use Bhasma of other gem stones such as tourmaline instead and obtain almost the same benefit. If gold Bhasma is beyond the reach of your pocketbook you can use pyrites (Suvarna Makshika, mentioned in the discussion on arthritis) Bhasma instead because it is also a Rasayana for Rasa Dhatu.

Even properly prepared Bhasmas can be dangerous if they are overused. Or, if the appropriate diet is not followed, they may have no effect. Vimalananda was once called upon to consult with a Maharaja. This ruler's court physicians, all well-trained Ayurvedic doctors, had been treating him for weeks with a Bhasma without any result. Vimalananda examined the prescription and found it to be correct, and then asked about diet. When he found that the Maharaja was still eating salt Vimalananda told him to stop it, and in a matter of days the disease disappeared.

Some minerals are not incinerated. Shilajit, a form of pitch which exudes from mountains in hot weather, is an ingredient in rejuvenating compounds such as Chandra Prabha, which is useful in many conditions including diabetes, obesity, and urinary tract complaints. It strengthens the immune system, regulates the menstrual cycle, and tones the male reproductive organs. Shilajit is also used dissolved with other herbs and honey in hot milk, to promote physical and mental strength and virility.

Since Bhasmas are still generally unavailable, some metals can be used in their pure forms. Bracelets of pure copper, for example, are indeed good for rheumatism, as folk wisdom in this country has had it for years, because the copper scrapes Ama away from the tissues. Such bracelets can be used only by V and K people, however, and not by Ps because copper is too hot for Ps. Copper or even gold may burn a P person's skin when worn. Also, if copper leaves a green discoloration on your skin it indicates that your system is already quite hot and acidic and needs no copper.

If you cannot wear your desired metal you can drink your water from a copper or a silver glass, or boil a piece of 24-carat gold in water for about half an hour and then take the resulting water in doses of 1 tsp. You can also put a piece of a purified metal on your photograph, or on a lock of your cut hair, to provide you with vibrations from the metal without introducing it physically into your body.

Indians traditionally insert a thin wire of 24-carat gold into a longitudinal hole in a whole calamus root, and rub the root clockwise into 1/2 tsp. of honey on a flat surface. 3 rubs is the dose for a child; 7 or more for an adult. In India this paste is given to a child from birth until 3 to 6 months of age to activate the immune system, which gold does better than anything else because it is so Sweet and so nourishing to all Dhatus.

Makaradhwaja

Vimalananda taught me about the power of gold by reminding me that it is mined with the help of cyanide. Because cyanide can dissolve gold it must have a deep affinity for the yellow metal. Gold is a highly concentrated Sweet, a powerful nutrient for body, mind, and aura. It is tonic and rejuvenating, and it is possible that the tonic and rejuvenating effects of such substances as yarrow, bamboo, almonds, and apricots may be due to the tiny amounts of cyanogens (substances which release cyanide) which they contain.

Larger doses of cyanide kill by interfering with cellular respiration, the release of energy caused by the combination of oxygen with various substances inside a cell. Cells die when their energy sources are cut off. Gold, and small doses of cyanide, presumably exert the opposite effect of making cellular respiration more efficient so that it yields more energy with less waste.

Everyone's aura tells a different story of immune preparedness, according to the sort of physical and mental Ama which is polluting the personality. Golden is the healthiest color for an aura. The most common Sanskrit word for gold, Suvarna, literally means "beautiful color." Gold is after all solidified sunrays, and intake of gold is sure to gild your aura, provided of course that you can digest it.

Gold by itself may be difficult to digest, especially if it so inflames your physical fire of digestion that you begin to overindulge yourself, ignoring your physical limits. It is best, therefore, to consume gold after it has been further digested—by mercury. Gold is mercury's food, and when it is administered with mercury, the likelihood of its being properly digested by the body improves dramatically.

Mercury is described as the semen of Lord Shiva. This means that mercury is the embodiment on the physical plane of the fire of transformation. It can provide tremendous Tejas to any organism, and can make that organism digest almost anything. Since mercury is semen, or Shukra, it is the ultimate aphrodisiac, the supreme virilizer. Semen is alive, full of Prana; mercury can provide Prana to the system. Since Shukra is the raw material from which Ojas is produced, mercury can create unlimited Ojas in an organism. Mercury provides the body with all three essentials for life—Prana, Tejas, and Ojas—and can therefore control all Three Doshas.

Even after purification mercury is too powerful to use in metallic form. It is most commonly reacted with sulfur to form black sulfide of mercury, which after heating becomes red sulfide of mercury. Sulfur is the menstrual blood of Shiva's wife Parvati, the only substance which can properly control mercury's tremendous power. Since sulfur is a form of Blood which can create other beings, it is as if sulfur acts as the womb in which the mercurial semen develops into the new child: Kajjali, black sulfide of mercury.

Sulfur's affinity for heavy metals has long been known. The active portion of BAL, the first drug developed to remove heavy metals from the body, is two sulfur atoms. Black sulfide of mercury is almost totally insoluble in either water or weak acids, and so the potential for poisoning by free mercury is very low. Red sulfide of mercury is slightly more soluble, but its potential for causing toxicity is also low. In fact, sulfide of mercury is used to help prevent toxicity from elemental mercury in industries, so its innate safety is recognized even today.

There is no disease which mercury cannot cure if it is properly prepared and used, say the texts. If improperly prepared or misused, there is no disease it cannot cause. No proof of the second half of the ancient saying is necessary; all of us know how poisonous mercury is. The first half of the saying has been proved over centuries of safe use of mercury in Ayurvedic medicines. Side effects of mercury may be derived from impurities like other heavy metals which are not removed before the mercury is processed, or may result from improper processing. Anyone who wants to use mercury for rejuvenation must be exceptionally careful about its source, and must be sure that it has been properly prepared. No one should ever try to prepare mercury for internal use without proper training!

The quantity of mercury in any one pill is very small thanks to the processing procedure known as Bhavana. In Bhavana, an herbal decoction or juice is mixed with the medicinal substance, and the resulting mixture is rubbed slowly in a mortar and pestle until it dries. The smooth, gentle, continuous motion provides a smooth, gentle vibration to the medicine, and the rubbing and grinding reduce its particle size, thus improving its effectiveness. Each Bhavana reduces the mercurial concentration of the finished product and potentizes it, in much the same way as homeopathic medicines are potentized.

The most renowned of all mercurial rejuvenators is Makaradhwaja, whose main ingredients are mercury, sulfur and gold. It regenerates vigor and vitality, improves immunity, and assists in body development by increasing metabolic activity. Makaradhwaja benefits all sorts of acute disease states, including especially respiratory ailments like cold, influenza, and pneumonia, and all sorts of chronic conditions, such as low blood pressure, general exhaustion and nervous or mental debility. It can keep the whole being alert and energetic well into old age.

The best forms of Makaradhwaja have gold leaf on the outer surface of the pill as well as gold within. The dose of Makaradhwaja is usually one pill once or twice a day, crushed and made into a paste with honey or Chyavanprash, and washed down with a cup of warm milk and saffron. This should be taken at least 1/2 hour before meals, and should be continued for 3 to 6 weeks. It is usually best to take Makaradhwaja, and other mercury-based rejuvenators, during the coldest season of the year so that their powerful innate fire does not increase Pitta. Two cycles of mercury-based medicine each year are sufficient for most people.

Other Rasayanas

Other mercury-based rejuvenators include:

Parpati - black sulfide of mercury prepared into a thick film. Parpati tones and enlivens the membrane lining the colon, improving its ability to absorb Prana from ingested food. Gold, mica, iron, copper, and herbs are added to some Parpati compounds to achieve specific therapeutic effects.

Lakshmi Vilasa Rasa - its main ingredients, beyond mercury sulfide, are gold, silver, mica, copper, tin, iron, pearls, and aconite. Its rejuvenating effect concentrates on the heart and lungs, and the Dhatus Rasa and Blood.

Vasanta Kusumakara Rasa - its main ingredients are almost the same as in Lakshmi Vilasa Rasa, but its effects differ because of different Bhavanas. Vasanta Kusumakara undergoes 35 or more Bhavanas of such varied substances as cow's milk, sugar cane juice, jasmine flower juice, sandalwood tea, and musk water. It improves the body's ability to digest Rasa, which makes it effective therapeutically in diabetes, heart disease, and consumption. It is a strong virilizer.

Suvarna Malini Vasanta - one of a class of three closely related compounds which act mainly on consumption, this contains gold, pearls, mercury sulfide, white pepper, and another form of mercury called Kharpara, which like both black and white pepper dries excessive secretions, especially in the respiratory tract. 21 Bhavanas of lime juice are then performed. This drying effect makes these compounds useful in all sorts of diseases of Rasa Dhatu, such as chronic bronchitis, pleurisy, fever, consumption, leucorrhea, and anemia. It enhances the vision, helps build strong fetuses, and helps eliminate poisons from the system. In spite of its drying effect, it can reverse weight and energy loss which occurs after a serious disease, or in old age.

Suvarna Raja Vangeshvara - although its color is metallic golden it contains no gold. Its main constituents are mercury, sulfur, and tin. Ammonium chloride is used as a flux, and the mixture is heated in a glass vial on a sand bath. In this instance the desired result drops to the bottom of the vial, suggesting a strong action on the lower parts of the body, which is indeed the case. Suvarna Raja Vangeshvara is most effective in loss of Shukra, as from frequent masturbation or wet dreams, and in conditions like consumption which result from loss of Shukra. Impotence and premature ejaculation also respond, as do certain forms of diabetes.

Smrti Sagara Rasa - this pill, named "Ocean of Memory," is one of several compounds which contain arsenic. Arsenic is essential to human nutrition in small amounts, and is found naturally in such foods as almonds, barley, carrots, corn, grapes, oats, pineapple and rice. It is used in Indian medicine mainly as a powerful invigorator. Arsenic's oxide is quite poisonous and is less commonly used than its sulfides. Smrti Sagara Rasa contains mercury sulfide, copper oxide, arsenic bisulfide, and arsenic trisulfide, and is processed with 21 Bhavanas each of calamus root tea and gotu kola juice, and one Bhavana of Jyotishmati oil. These herbs are all well-known brain tonics. There is just sufficient arsenic in these pills to gently stimulate the memory.

Hema Garbha - containing mercury sulfide, gold, and copper oxide, this medicine is simmered in liquefied sulfur in an earthenware crucible, and made into a stick which is rubbed into a paste with honey on a stone and given sublingually when needed for extreme Vata disturbance like coma. It is a powerful rejuvenator and heart tonic.

These are only a few of the many Ayurvedic rejuvenators available. It is impossible to overstate the dangers inherent in self-dosing yourself with any of these substances. Never experiment with any of these substances on your own; consume them only under the direct supervision of a qualified Ayurvedic physician.

Seasons

A Sufi from Bombay once gave me his prescription for good health. "Most of the time," he said, "I live a strict life, and always eat at home.

But once a month I make it a point to go to a restaurant and eat a good meal. Eating regularly in restaurants is not healthy, I know, but at least once a month it is good to do so, to expose your system to all the diseases which are prevalent in the community. Then your immune system is prepared for anything that might otherwise sneak up on you unawares."

This is good advice. It is unwise to try to live too pure a life nowadays. There are too many pollutants around us, in our air, water and food, for us to be totally pristine. And even if you thoroughly purify yourself today, the environment will begin to pollute you again tomorrow. Purification cannot be done once and then forgotten about. Ayurveda mandates regular purification for preventative maintenance, followed by rejuvenation to counteract the recurrent destabilizations of life.

We may try to insulate ourselves from the influence of external forces with humidifiers, air conditioners and central heaters, but we are exposed to the environment every time we leave our cocoons. This continual reorientation causes continual stress. In attempting to create a standard year-round environment we have engineered instead a year-round source of stress.

All constitutional weaknesses are strongly influenced by time. Vata-caused problems, for example, always worsen "when clouds fill the sky," much as our old timers claim that the appearance of aches and pains in their rheumatic joints forecasts a storm. Any change of weather is likely to disturb Vata, since Vata is aggravated by change, but each constitution is affected differently during each season. "Season" includes all sorts of time cycles:

V predominates - after eating before digestion begins
during the pre-dawn and late afternoon hours
during autumn and early winter
in old age

P predominates - during digestion
at midday and midnight
during summer
in middle age

K predominates - after digestion, during assimilation
at daybreak and nightfall
during late winter and spring
in childhood and youth

A V person naturally finds it more difficult to maintain balance when V predominates in a season; likewise for P and K. Autumn is often the worst season for Vs because the weather is most changeable then, and because wind storms like hurricanes and tornados are prevalent. V people should not begin major new projects in the fall, and even if they bend their dietary and lifestyle rules during the rest of the year they should renew their discipline in autumn, to maintain harmony in all areas of their lives. Ps must be strictest with themselves during summer, or whenever else it is exceedingly hot. K people most need discipline in spring, when the snow melts and the sap runs in Nature, and the Kapha flows in the body.

Everyone must be alert, however, to prevent imbalance during the "joints" between these seasons, the periods when one season is changing into another and the "weather" is not sure itself which season it belongs to. This external confusion in Nature is mirrored by internal confusion in the organism. Spring fever, for example, can strike anyone, and is due to the inertia carried by the powerful flow of Kapha which happens at the end of winter.

Regular purification can control this. Since Kapha predominates in the spring, removal of excess Kapha when winter has died but spring has not yet quite been born can prevent diseases due to Kapha accumulation. Excess Pitta should be eliminated in the interim between spring and summer, and excess Vata between summer and fall.

India's Rishis created festivals and traditions to encourage everyone to remember to change their diets and habits as the seasons changed. For example, on the day after the New Moon nearest the vernal equinox people in Western India always eat a few neem leaves early in the morning before consuming anything else. They say that in this way there will be no bitterness during the rest of the year; the hidden meaning is that there need be no Bitterness due to disease if neem or another Bitter substance is used then to control Kapha, which is predominant then, and Pitta, which acculumates then becomes predominant as the weather warms up.

According to the Indian calendar the sun moves into Capricorn on January 14. You must eat sesame seeds and jaggery (solidified sugar cane juice) on this day so that you will speak sweetly for the rest of the year. Sesame seeds, especially the black variety, are nourishing and virilizing but difficult to digest. Since the body's digestive fire is strongest in the winter, when extra food is needed to keep warm, consumption of black sesame seeds and jaggery then helps preserve the body's strength. This makes all its sense organs better able to function ("speak") efficiently ("sweetly") during the coming months of aggravated Doshas. Time is an important factor in the life of every mortal, and living according to Nature's time is the only way to remain healthy.

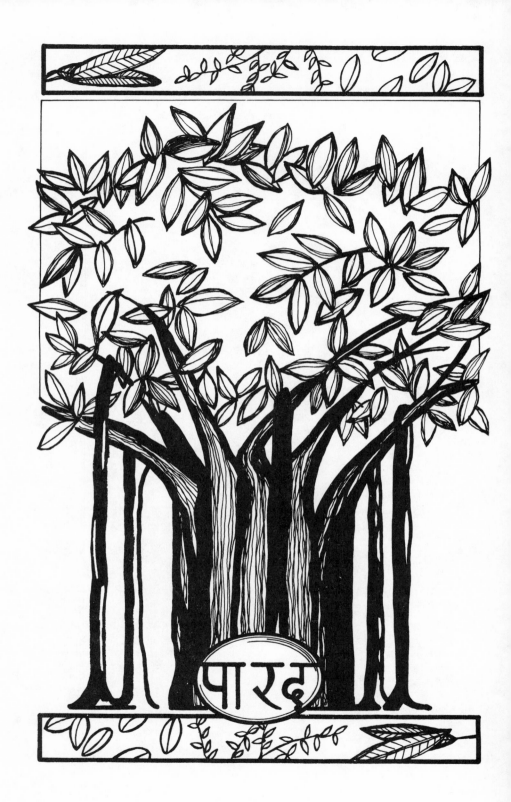

Chapter Nine
Beyond Ayurveda

Immortality

Ahamkara uses body and mind for her gratification as long as she can, but even with good rejuvenation the organism eventually wears out. Dependence on the external universe for any kind of nourishment—physical, mental, emotional, or spiritual—causes wear and tear. Mind, senses and spirit cannot be satisfied by "bread alone"; they must feel *prasanna*, or "satisfied," to be healthy. As long as they believe that they need sensory gratification to be satisfied they will maintain their external orientation, searching the outside world for gratification.

Mind and spirit need not be wholly dependent on the body. For example, 300 out of 600 individuals with hydrocephalus, a condition in which 95% of the volume of the skull is filled with cerebro-spinal fluid instead of brain tissue, were found to have IQs greater than 100, indicating above average intelligence. If the mind can function without most of its brain it should also be able to function without many of the other things we think it requires. The Rishis understood this, and because they wanted to go beyond the limitations of time they realized that reliance on external sustenance makes an individual subject to time.

They also knew that each season has its own Taste, which permeates the food, water and air available to us during that season. Since Taste influences emotion, and since mortals are dependent on external sources of Rasa, they realized that their mental balance was also dependent on the influences of the seasonal changes of the environment.

They therefore restricted themselves first to roots and fruits, then to milk, then to water, and finally solely to air, to eliminate the negative physical and mental effects of all physical food. They learned how to obtain their Prana from the air, and how to create all Dhatus and ultimately even Ojas directly from this Prana with the help of the powerful Tejas enkindled in them by their spiritual austerities. This permitted them to escape from the influence of external Rasa, and made them immortal.

An immortal does not need to eat physical food because his or her organism can create all Six Tastes internally, within itself, in the proper proportions needed for Ahamkara's self-expression. Immortality is true freedom, freedom from all limitations. A mortal cannot simply decide one day to do without food altogether; the system has to be adapted to it.

The food we eat provides us a very crude form of Prana. That Prana which comes in with each breath through the nostrils is much finer, but is still crude compared to that which can be obtained through the eyes by such processes as Trataka, staring at flames or the sun. The supreme form of Prana is that which is imbibed by the mind directly from the universe telepathically, without the interposition of any sense organ. The subtler forms of Prana are much Sweeter than Prana from normal sources. They require little digestion, satiate body and mind more profoundly, and can be imbibed only through internal concentration. Thus the Yogis speak of enjoying Jnanamrtam Bhojanam, "the nectar of knowledge for sustenance."

Even those of us who lack the perfect internal concentration to obtain these finer forms of Prana can obtain refined Prana from mercury. One interpretation of the word "Rasayana" is "the Path of Mercury." Rasashastra, the "Science of Rasa," is the art of purifying and controlling mercury to utilize its power to evaporate the effects of ageing. Crude mercury cannot do this; it is far too poisonous. After preliminary purifications, Prana is added to crude mercury and it is brought to life. It is then awakened, instructed, fed, bound, swooned, and sacrificed. These refining processes are called Samskaras.

The word Samskara is closely related to the word Sanskrit, which is actually spelled Samskrta, "that which has undergone Samskaras." Sanskrit is not an ordinary language, one which evolved by trial and error over centuries of mass mispronunciation. Sanskrit is a product of phonetic engineering. Each of its words has a vibratory meaning in addition to its overt meaning. This is why Sanskrit is called a Mantric language, a language in which each word is a Mantra. A Mantra is a group of sounds which when pronounced in a certain way creates a certain vibration both in the brain and body of the pronouncer, and on anything into which the pronouncer chooses to direct the vibration.

Just as food can carry prayer or hatred into the system, a Mantra's vibration can be carried on any substance, even water, into the body. Because Mantras are much more subtle than physical fire and grinding, Mantrically-prepared medicines exert a profounder effect on the whole organism than ordinary medicines can. Samskaras on mercury were originally performed with both herbs and Mantras, and the medicines thus produced were exponentially more powerful than are today's commercially prepared medicines whose Samskaras are performed with herbs alone.

One Sanskrit word for mercury is Parada, that which carries you to the far shore of existence and makes you immortal. It is also called Rasa, because it has a perfect complement of Six Tastes. Yogis say that while herbs can keep you alive 400 to 500 years mercury can keep you alive forever, if you understand the discipline and restrictions behind its use. Mercury is the sole metal or mineral which can actually be brought to life. The alchemist creates life in mercury and then takes it again; he sacrifices the mercury to obtain its Prana.

Sacrifice

External alchemy developed from the internal alchemy of Tantra, and like all else in the Vedic universe it is rooted in the concept of sacrifice. The Cosmic Being sacrificed His own body; each part developed into an aspect of the universe. An immortal emulates the Cosmic Being. After Ahamkara's nutrition is guaranteed, an immortal permits the borders of self to dissolve and allows Nature to direct his or her every move. Ahamkara has to eat, and Nature is always willing to provide food to all Her children. She sacrifices Herself for Herself. To repay the debt this sacrifice incurs the immortal offers all action as a sacrifice to Her, to offer Her nourishment and to remedy the imbalances Her other children cause in Her. Immortals work to preserve the health of the body politic.

Ahamkara is addicted to food. Most of us are addicted to physical food; saints and sages eliminate ordinary addictions and addict themselves to God. Addiction is the basis for all disorder and disharmony, and addiction to God is the only permanent cure. Addiction to God eliminates all possibility of interference from other beings, because body, mind and spirit are all concentrated on the same object. Since all diseases are due to alien influences, you become disease-free. Even if you are not yet immortal, transferring your addictions to God can transform your existence.

Shiva, Vishnu and all the other Indian deities are cosmic forces. The Rishis assigned them personalities based on the emotions they create within us. A deity's emotion-personality is just like the Taste-personality which a food or a medicine displays. If you know how to adapt it to your condition, you can make use of its tastes or emotions to balance your system. Herbs and minerals are also cosmic forces, but they are limited by being physical. A deity's personality comes much closer to being unlimited.

For example, Krishna, who is an aspect of Vishnu, is Sweetness personified. Everything Krishna touches becomes Sweet, or "Madhura," because Krishna Himself is "Madhu," the unlimited, unqualified cosmic Sweetness. Anyone who makes proper use of Krishna's Mantra, even someone who doesn't believe in deities and doubts Krishna's history, can drink from the bottomless well of permanently satisfying Sweetness which Krishna personifies.

The Vedic, Puranic, and Tantric spiritual disciplines, which are wrongly referred to collectively as the Hindu religion, present a com-

bined physical and mental approach to enhanced spiritual development.
Specific herbs have been associated with specific deities for millennia:
wood apple with Shiva and Lakshmi, coconut with Lakshmi, holy basil
with Vishnu, Bermuda grass with Ganesha, and so on. These herbs give
physical, mental, and spiritual benefits to devotees who use them properly.

For example, Bermuda grass controls blood sugar in elephants, who
love to eat Sweet food, and can do the same for humans who use it.
When this Bermuda grass is sacrificed to Ganesha before use its medical effect is multiplied manyfold.

Or consider the ritual worship known as the Satya Narayana Puja,
in which 1000 leaves of holy basil are offered to Vishnu. The leaves are
collected after being offered with Mantras, and their juice is extracted
and administered. Shira, a preparation of wheat groats cooked in ghee,
is eaten as food. The Tulasi juice and the Shira work together to provide the rejuvenating effect: the Tulasi enkindles all the digestive fires,
and the Shira provides nourishment for these enkindled fires to digest.

Most people today in India perform this ritual mechanically, unaware
of its true significance. Vishnu is the Preserver, the cosmic force which
perpetuates life, and the holy basil is one of Vishnu's wives, one of the
forces Vishnu uses to preserve life. This suggests that Tulasi (holy basil)
is one of the best of all substances for preserving life.

The Satya Narayana Puja, at one level of meaning, is a process of
potentizing Tulasi leaves to increase their life-extending effects so they
can act as a rejuvenator for the individual who consumes them. This
potentiation is comparable to the potentiation provided by Bhavana and
incineration, but Mantras are used solely instead of any physical processing. The Satya Narayana Puja was written by the Rishis, who in-
tuited both Tulasi's qualities and the appropriate sounds which could
enhance these qualities.

Even if you are a Christian or a Muslim, or you oppose paganism for
some other reason, you can still use the Satya Narayana Puja to improve
your physical health. Faith in the ritual's esoteric significance enhances
its effects, but some effect will be produced no matter what you think
of it, if the Mantras are pronounced correctly. Potentiation by Mantra is
as scientific as any other form of potentiation, though it is much more
subtle. Mantras are impersonal bundles of power, which are more comprehensible to us when we make use of the personalities the Rishis have
provided for us. Meditation on a cosmic personality, concentrating and
directing its force into you, metamorphosizes your own personality to
resemble your object of concentration.

Kundalini

You can use mercury as a rejuvenator even if you cannot bring your-self to believe that it is Lord Shiva's semen. To walk the path of mer-cury and get the most you can out of it, though, there is no substitute for the worship of Shiva. Lord Shiva dwells in every human being, deep in the brain. He is pure, unalloyed consciousness. True immortality is possible only when your personal Shiva has complete control over His Shakti, or power, your Ahamkara. One of Shiva's aspects is named Mahakala, Infinite Time. As long as a human remains in ordinary time-bound mundane consciousness, this Ahamkara-Shakti, known as Kun-dalini, identifies continually with the body. Human life exists only because the Kundalini deludes herself into believing that she and the limited body-mind personality are identical.

When Kundalini is completely awakened, she realizes that she is Shiva's Shakti. Any human who has not already undergone strenuous penance will be transported beyond normal mundane time into infinity by this experience. In such circumstances the body cannot continue to exist, because Kundalini will immediately forget it and will remember Shiva. She sacrifices her identity to Him, undergoing instant enlighten-ment in the process.

If like the Yogis you have used the Shiva-consciousness to prepare your physical, mental and spiritual being for this tremendous evolution-ary experience, there is a chance that you will be able to retain your body at least for a time. If you have become immortal you can keep your body forever, and can instruct your Kundalini to identify with it, or to forget it and identify with Shiva, at your whim. This is absolute health, total control of Ahamkara and its immune defenses.

Many people follow spiritual disciplines, hoping to become enlightened through meditation and other austerities. Most of these people do so with only a hazy knowledge of physical and mental phys-iology; very few of them know anything at all about Ayurveda. Some-times they experiment with powers like Kundalini of which they know little. Like all other powerful medicines, Kundalini can cure all ailments when properly approached, and can cause all ailments when improp-erly employed.

If you are physically and mentally unprepared for this forcible rip-ping away of Ahamkara from its safe haven in your limited human body with its attendant personality, you will suffer severe, permanent physi-cal and psychic damage. The "Kundalini crisis," a disease in which Kun-dalini's power is unleashed in an unprepared organism, is a serious disorder because like cancer it is a direct assault on personality.

If the personality tries to resist Kundalini's arousal a crisis occurs. A fully-awakened Kundalini in an unprepared individual forgets the body entirely, and the organism dies. This process is much like transmitting millions of volts of electricity over a line meant to handle 110 volts. The line instantly vaporizes into its constituent atoms, and no part of it remains intact. This is why Shiva is called the god of death, and why you must make Shiva your adviser if you hope to awaken Kundalini without destroying yourself in the process.

If Kundalini is only partially awakened, however, when she begins to move through untested nervous and endocrine systems, those systems will collapse, or blow out. If you send 220 volts over a 110 volt line, the insulation will burn through and the line may melt in a few places. Though its essential integrity remains it cannot function without repair. In an unprepared human body a Kundalini surge burns the insulation off the nervous system and melts some of the body's endocrine controls. Life remains, but it is unbalanced.

In V types, or in people afflicted with Vata disturbances, Kundalini hits with the force of a hurricane or a tornado. In P types and in those with aggravated Pitta, Kundalini envelops the victim in flames. K types may resist longer, but as the crisis develops they too tumble into the fire or are buffeted by the gale. When the body is full of Ama, this wind blows Ama to all parts of the body, and the fire cooks the Ama into virulent poison.

This is enough for most people: they realize that the danger involved in spiritual advancement is the danger of personality extinction. The fear of death of the limited identity is at the base of a Kundalini crisis. The shock of the knowledge of impending personality disintegration terrifies their unprepared personalities into retreat. Unfortunately, there is no retreat. You can't go home again, once your home has been demolished by a Kundalini earthquake. Many sufferers from this Shakti blowout exist in limbo, unable to go forward or backward, immobilized by the profundity of their fear.

The Kundalini crisis feels uncontrollable to its victims because it is a disorder of Ahamkara herself, a disorder which threatens the individual's "I-forming" capability. When your personality is undergoing dissolution, how can it properly control anything?

In no other disease is the axiom "prevention is better than cure" more apropos. Once an individual is in the throes of a Kundalini crisis there is no quick remedy, no simple solution, because there is no physical procedure which can reverse the energy flow and recoil the Serpent. Acupuncture can help, as can Yogic breathing techniques and Ayurvedic massage, but all these therapies are merely symptomatic. You should certainly seek professional help if Kundalini is your concern, but there is no turning back from her. You must adapt or perish.

The Ayurvedic texts state that disease first entered the world when Shiva destroyed the sacrifice of Daksha. Daksha was a great Yogi, a being so spiritually advanced that the Rishis themselves officiated at his sacrifice. Shiva was forced to destroy the sacrifice because Daksha was unwilling to relinquish his attachment to his achievements. This story has a moral for everyone who works with Kundalini, because the Shiva who is within each one of us can destroy all achievements and create all diseases unless our sacrifice is unselfish.

Daksha believed he was powerful enough to control Kundalini with his own personality, but he learned to his dismay that only Shiva's personality is strong enough to provide Kundalini boundaries and direction. Because Kundalini is also the sexual energy, the story of the destruction of Daksha's sacrifice is also the story of the sexual act as practiced by ordinary humans. Permitting themselves to believe that they are in complete control they enjoy sexual excitation until orgasm, when all the energy they had mobilized is suddenly projected outward. This violent cycle of manifestation and loss of energy inevitably increases Vata, and thus disease, in the organism. Control of Kundalini is possible only through control of sexual response.

Kundalini forcibly peels away puny human limitations and propels one toward a truly unlimited existence. The pineal gland is involved at this stage of personal transmutation. It is the pineal which controls the conversion of Shukra, the male and female sex secretions, the ultimate physical expressions of the creative Ahamkara, into Ojas, which forms the aura. Ahamkara must make a leap of faith for this process to succeed. She must be willing to sacrifice part of herself, part of her own existence, in order to go beyond herself and, paradoxically, to perpetuate herself. The concept of sacrifice is central to the Vedas because without sacrifice there is no transcendence, no "getting beyond yourself" into a new realm of existence.

Darkness and Light

Modern scientists are beginning to study melatonin, one of the pineal's chief hormones. It seems to control our circadian rhythms, those internal seasonal clocks which determine whether we are "morning" or "night" people, and whether winter makes us exalted or depressed. These rhythms are disrupted by our artificially created time sense, which created activities such as shift work, and by long-distance jet travel, activities which disturb our natural routine of day and night.

Melatonin helps determine how much "darkness" or "light" is present in an individual organism. It also helps determine our Tastes, both in terms of food preferences and psychological moods. Depression and other psychological disorders can be due to too much melatonin, which is usually due to insufficient exposure to light. In fact light stimulation has been shown to improve such conditions as manic depression, schizophrenia, migraines, and anorexia. More sunlight on your skin and in your eyes means increased sex drive and fertility as melatonin decreases.

Consider one very interesting fact: you can drink more alcohol at night in a dark corner than you can during the day, or in a well-lighted place. Alcohol powerfully aggrandizes Ahamkara. She weakens and loses all her introspection under alcohol's influence, and proceeds to satisfy all her desires without the interference of conscience or qualm. Alcoholism seems to be aggravated by high melatonin levels. When the pineal is properly stimulated by light, it reduces egotism; in the darkness, the pineal stimulates selfishness. Since Ojas is produced by sacrifice, light promotes the production of Ojas; darkness, because it encourages self-indulgence, retards Ojas production.

Though no scientist has yet been able to isolate Ojas, it is surely the "light" counterpart of "dark" melatonin. Melatonin is the shadow, produced when Ahamkara tries to interpose herself between the individual and the pure perception of reality. Ojas allows the light of reality to flood the organism without obstruction. To be led "from darkness into light," from higher to lower melatonin production, is essential if one is to be led "from untruth into truth," from the untruth of selfish Ahamkara-centered sensory indulgence to the truth of Ojas-producing Shukra sacrifice. Then only, when Ojas is at its zenith, can one be led "from mortality into immortality."

Tarpana

There is no permanent physical or mental cure for constitutional weaknesses. Once you have identified yourself as a V, P, or K type, or as a combination of two of these, you are stuck with that constitution, and all its benefits and defects, until you die. There are only two ways to escape. One way of escape is open to you if you are a spiritual aspirant, and follow strict spiritual disciplines. Under such controlled conditions there will be little occasion for your constitution to display itself. It will not change, but it will not disturb you. The other way involves the ancient ritual of Tarpana. Related to the Sanskrit word Trpti, which means satiation or satisfaction, Tarpana is a process of gratifying your ancestors.

There is a Law of Nature known as the Bija Vrksha Nyaya: the Law of Seed and Tree. Your seeds are your genes and chromosomes, the essence of your parents' germ plasm. You are the tree, the product of those seeds. Half your genes come from one parent, and half from the other. No matter how far you try to distance yourself from your parents, in space, time, or interaction, your genes and their genes are identical, and resonate with one another. Your parents' emotions are bound to resonate with your emotions, no matter how far distant you may be from them, because of this fundamental identity. This is why a certain telepathic communication sometimes exists between parent and child.

Because your parents' genes originated in your grandparents, your emotions will be influenced by their emotions, and by the emotions of your great-grandparents, and so on, back at least seven generations. Even though most of your ancestors are already dead the subtle effects of their personalities remain in your genetic environment and continue to affect you.

Homeopathic medicine discusses miasms, inherited weaknesses which are passed down from generation to generation in a family. These inherited weaknesses are referred to in Sanskrit as Kutumba Dosha, "faults in the family." Ayurvedic rejuvenation works on the physical manifestations of these faults. Tarpana works more deeply, reducing the emotional charges which have accumulated in you as a result of the activities of your forebears.

Suppose one of your ancestors was overly fond of eating, so fond that he or she fantasized about food all day long. All cravings are forms of energy, which are broadcast into the Ether with every thought. Some of these thoughts will be rational and sensible, but many will be obsessive. You, who are permanently tuned to your ancestors' wavelengths, automatically receive these subtle broadcasts, which will induce you to become obsessive about food if you are susceptible to them.

Anyone who is really obsessive about food is likely to be thinking of food at the moment of death. This final broadcast message is more powerful than all those which went before, because it is transmitted with all the anguish of an unfillable desire. Because of the power behind this desire, and the fact that the individual whose rational mind could partly negate it no longer exists, this last wish affects you much more powerfully than any living wishes can.

Tarpana enables you to negate these desires. Once they are gone, the pressure on your genes to make you obsessive about food eases, and your diet and habits can induce other of your genes to begin to function, which changes your emotional climate. As long as these unseen influences continue to affect you no amount of diet or routine can ever eliminate them because they do not strike at the source. 99% of human and chimpanzee genes are identical; the differences between the two species occur because some genes are expressed more than others. You are your own creator, ceaselessly creating yourself from your own genes with the help of your physical and mental food and habits.

The traditional ritual of Tarpana is complex, but its essence is simple. It is much like the All Soul's Day tradition, when people visit their relatives in the cemetery. In preparation, consider what one food item your parent or grandparent was fondest of. Maybe it is the apple strudel your grandmother used to bake, or the ale your father used to drink. That food will act as a vehicle for your emotion.

Sit comfortably facing south and visualize your dead ancestors, one by one, as far back as you can remember. Make each one sit in front of you. Telling them you want to help release them from any residual earthly desires they might have, offer them a spoonful of water, a spoonful of milk, and a spoonful of sesame seeds, preferably the black variety. These offerings are the same for everyone.

Then offer a little of the special item, with the heartfelt wish that this will satisfy any residual cravings and allow that individual, wherever he or she is, to continue with their own progression towards greater integration and clarity. You then request them to return whence they came, and feed the food you have offered to an animal, or put it into a river or the ocean. It is good to repeat this annually, preferably on the same New Moon Day each year. The best days for Tarpana are New Moon Days, especially those which fall in September.

You need not even believe in reincarnation, or even life after death, to perform Tarpana. Your parents and grandparents are still alive inside you, in your genes. You are simply projecting a part of your personality, contacting it, and requesting it to be pleased with you and to relinquish any inappropriate influence it may have over you. This visualization releases you from any unhealthy psychological habits you may have as a result of the influence of these previous beings who also shared your genes, and of the images you have of those beings.

Tarpana is especially important for ancestors you knew personally. If you loved them, you show them your love in the only way remaining to you, by remembering them and offering part of yourself to them as a token of your love. If your relationship with them was marred by negative emotions, Tarpana allows you to forgive them, to heal the relationship by sacrificing your negativity and offering them the healing power of your love. Thankfulness for the genes which have given you life, and forgiveness for those genes which have limited your existence, transport the sacrifice to its intended target.

If you are convinced that this procedure can actually help eliminate any negativity remaining between you and the image you hold of your ancestor, it will. Faith is essential for it to work; you must make your offering with complete sincerity. Faith can truly make you whole.

Faith can make our society whole as well. Tarpana is important to all of us who have forgotten our roots. It recreates the bond which should exist between us and our ancestors. Indian tradition regards Tarpana as a duty which every child must perform for its parents. When we accept this responsibility we relinquish forgetfulness. Tarpana is an act of remembrance which solidifies the link between the generations. By opening ourselves to our ancestral influences and forgiving our forebears their imperfections, we open ourselves to their accumulated wisdom, which can cement our culture together.

Conclusion

Unless you are already immortal, your health is a dynamic condition, not a permanent state. There is no limit to the harmony possible in you, and no limit to the harmony you can create around yourself. The ultimate aim is true freedom, freedom from reliance on the external world, which can come only when you make yourself a balanced, self-sustaining cosmos. None of us who are mortal are truly free; we are all obliged to purchase our limited freedom with eternal vigilance.

We are limited by our concepts of limitation. Restructuring of our belief systems is the key to permitting ourselves unlimited personal development. If we can learn to walk on fire without being burned we can also learn to eliminate side-effects from therapy with powerful drugs and heal surgical wounds quickly. Ayurveda and its sister sciences provide directions for our attempts to enter into a sincere, bonded relationship with Nature, Who is the source of faith and forgiveness. Filled with faith, we can move mountains.

Our task on this imperfect planet is to work continuously towards relative perfection. The beginning of world perfection is self-perfection. In the words of the song, "Let there be peace on earth, and let it begin with me." Self-perfection requires self-peace, which begins with elimination of your physical, mental, and emotional limitations. Understanding, honesty, acceptance, forgiveness and compassion are your tools for self-development. Nature is forgiveness incarnate, and all healing comes from Nature.

Use your Doshas to help you. A healthy person uses the V mode to obtain original, creative ideas, moves into the P mode to engineer the theory into a plan for actualizing it, and employs the K mode to follow through on the plan. Healthy people are well-rounded. Instead of berating yourself for your imperfections, overcome them with the help of your inner light.

If you are a V person you must forgive yourself for being chaotic, for sometimes being so hyperactive that you neglect what needs to be done. If you are a P person you must accept your innate impatience with other people and with yourself. You must never let the fact of this impatience interfere with your process of harmonizing yourself and your surroundings. If you are a K person you must forgive yourself your complacency and be willing to move beyond it.

If you are already ill you must be able to forgive your disease. You must forgive Ahamkara for being dependent on Fat for love if you are overweight. If you have arthritis you must forgive yourself for creating an alien servant to stiffen your joints for you. If cancer has invaded you Ahamkara must be forgiven for being so confused that she has empowered another identity to try to force her into confronting her problems. Forgiveness permits you to break free from all the things you have bitten off, chewed up and swallowed that you cannot digest. You can leave them behind you, and create a new self-image. Give a new image to Ahamkara to identify with, and she can create a healthy organism for you.

The prayer below can be your covenant with the universe. You offer yourself as an instrument to try to make the world a better place through whatever efforts, however meager. When you say it sincerely, Nature will in return offer Her powers to heal you and your environment:

May everyone be happy

May everyone be healthy

May everything be holy

May there never be disharmony of any kind, anywhere!

This is the message of Ayurveda.

For further information on Ayurveda and how to order the Ayurvedic Home Study Course please contact:

The Ayurvedic Institute
P.O. Box 23445
Albuquerque, NM 87192-1445

For Ayurvedic products unavailable elsewhere:

Kanak
P.O. Box 13653
Albuquerque, NM 87192-3653

APPENDIX

Khichadi - Split Mung Beans and Rice

This preparation, a common staple food for many Indians, is also a purifying, balancing diet suitable for almost everyone. It is ideal for those with poor digestion or assimilation because it is easy to digest and also assists in eliminating toxins from the system.

2 cups rice, preferably Indian basmati rice
1 cup split mung beans (called "mung dal" in Indian grocery stores)
8 to 12 cups water, depending on how liquid you want the final product to be
2 Tbsp. ghee (clarified butter)
1 tsp. ground cumin
1 scant tsp. ground coriander seed
1/4 to 1/2 tsp. turmeric powder
3 to 5 whole cardamom pods
1 to 2 tsp. of powdered ginger
pinch salt or powdered kelp
pinch asafoetida powder

If you are unable to locate an Indian grocery store you can substitute sprouted mung beans for the split variety. Wash off the green seed covers which split when the beans sprout. One part beans to two parts rice is the standard proportion. Those individuals with malfunctioning digestions may choose to reduce the proportion of beans to rice to 1:3, or even less. Those with stronger digestions may increase the proportion to 1:1 if they so desire.

Wash the beans and rice and soak them separately in an excess of water for at least an hour. Thereafter discard the soak water, mix the beans and rice together and rinse them with fresh water.

Heat gently 2 Tbsp. of ghee. While heating, add the cumin, coriander, turmeric and asafoetida. Saute these spices lightly in the ghee, until they are just browned but before they blacken, and add the mung beans and rice, stirring vigorously for about a minute so that some of the spices will be absorbed. Then add water, ginger, cardamom and salt or kelp, bring to a slow boil, cover, and cook until the individual grains are completely soft. Serve with yogurt for V types and extra ghee for P people. K individuals should use more spices and less water. This amount will serve five or six people.

As digestion improves the amount of spices may be increased, and onion, garlic, daikon radish, and other root vegetables may be added to the mixture before cooking begins.

Glossary

Ahamkara - literally, the "I-former." Ahamkara is that force which identifies herself with an individual body, mind and spirit and permits them to exist together as a living being. She is feminine because she is a portion of the creative power of Mother Nature. Uncontrolled, Ahamkara may, by identifying with objects which are external to the individual, create unhealthy dependencies and addictions.

Ama - a general term for internal toxins produced by improper metabolic functioning.

Amalaki - *Emblica officinalis*, the Indian gooseberry, which is the part of Triphala which best controls Pitta. It is the main ingredient in the rejuvenating jam known as Chyvanprash.

Anabolism - the force which causes the body to grow and develop.

Antibody - a protein created by the body which is specific to a particular antigen and helps remove that antigen from the system.

Antigen - any substance which the body recognizes as foreign to it and reacts to by production of an antibody.

Aura - the subtle energy field which pervades and surrounds the human body. The aura is produced by ojas.

Bhasma - literally "ash," a Bhasma is a metal or mineral incinerated after a given number of Bhavanas and used for therapeutic purposes.

Bhavana - a process for enhancing the qualities of a substance; it is most often performed with a mortar and pestle.

Bibhitaki - *Terminalia bellerica*, the ingredient in Triphala which best controls Kapha.

Brahmacharya - literally "walking with the Creator," it is used to indicate some degree of sexual restraint for purposes of physical, mental and spiritual health.

Catabolism - the force which breaks down and consumes body tissues.

Chyvanprash - a rejuvenating jam whose main ingredient is the Amalaki fruit.

Dhatu - literally, "that which supports the body." A Dhatu is one of the seven body tissues which when well-nourished nourish Ahamkara

Dosha - literally "fault" or "mistake," a Dosha is one of the three forces which bind the Five Great Elements down into living flesh. They are Vata, Pitta, and Kapha.

Emmenagogue - a substance which helps initiate menstrual flow.

Endometrium - the lining of the womb which is replaced monthly. It acts as a bed for the zygote should a woman become pregnant, and is sloughed during menstruation if she does not.

Ganesha - the gentle elephant-headed deity of India who removes obstacles from the way of his devotees.

Ghee - clarified butter, prepared by simmering unsalted butter on lowest possible heat until all the water boils off and then straining out the milk solids. The purified fat remaining is the ghee.

Guduchi - *Tinospora cordifolia*, a vine from which a Bitter white powder is extracted which is regarded as one of the best of Bitter tonics in Ayurveda.

Guggulu - *Commiphora mukul*, a gum or resin from a tree native to India and Pakistan which is used in combination with other herbs to scrape Ama from Fat, Flesh, and Bone.

Haritaki - *Terminalia chebula*, the ingredient in Triphala which best controls Vata.

Lakshmi - the cosmic power of physical abundance and wealth.

Laxation - the use of mild to medium laxatives to encourage Pitta and Kapha to flow freely from the system.

Madhura - Sweet which must first be digested, as opposed to Madhu, Sweet which is predigested, like honey.

Madhuvinashini - *Gymnema sylvestre*, a leaf which when chewed temporarily removes the tongue's ability to taste Sweet, and reduces its ability to taste Bitter (Madhu "Sweet" + Vinashini "Destroyer").

Neem - *Azadirachta indica*, a tropical tree whose parts are very Bitter. It is used mainly in disorders of the skin and the liver.

Ojas - a hormone-like substance which is derived from Shukra. It produces the aura, transmits energy from mind to body, and controls immunity.

Panchakarma - the Five Purification Methods, used to rid the body of excess Doshas. They are: enema, purgation, emesis, nasal medication and bloodletting.

Parada - "that which takes you beyond mortality," the metal mercury.

Pippali - *Piper longum* or long pepper, a cousin of black pepper used mainly for strengthening the respiratory tract, for improving the body's ability to utilize nourishment, and as an aphrodisiac.

Prajnaparadha - literally "crime against wisdom," it signifies that perversity of mind which willfully acts in a way known to be unhealthy.

Prakruti - literally, "first action." Prakruti in Ayurveda refers to an individual's inherent "nature," the inborn tendencies which influence consciousness and activity. Prakruti determines which response your body or mind first displays to a stress.

Prana - the life force, called ki or chi in Oriental medicine.

Prasanna - "satisfied." Mind, senses and soul are healthy only when they are Prasanna.

Prinana - the function of Rasa Dhatu, the first of the Dhatus. Prinana provides the body satisfaction like that obtained through romantic love.

Purgation - the use of medium to strong laxatives to expel excess Pitta or Kapha from the system.

Rajas - the cosmic force of activity. Excess Rajas causes the mind to become overactive and unstable.

Rasa - (1) taste, especially the Six Tastes of Ayurveda, and the emotions derived therefrom. (2) the first Dhatu, also called chyle or plasma, analogous to the sap of plants. (3) semen (Shukra), especially that of Lord Shiva, and by extension the metal mercury.

Rishi - a Seer; an immortal being able to perceive hidden realities and manifest those realities in a way comprehensible to humans. The ancient Rishis created Ayurveda in this way out of compassion for the sufferings of humanity.

Samskara - a conditioning process. Children are raised by imparting cultural Samskaras to them, and mercury is prepared for use in medicine with the help of physical Samskaras.

Sanga Dosha - the detrimental effect on one's own consciousness experienced when one associates with selfish, unbalanced people.

Satsanga - literally, "association with the good," the act of spending one's time with someone more integrated. Satsanga actively improves one's own personality intergration.

Sattva - the cosmic force of equilibrium, which is the normal balanced state of a healthy mind.

Shakti - power or energy, described as female in the ancient texts.

Shiva - the embodiment of cosmic consciousness; the god of death Who eventually rescues the individual Ahamkara from self-identifying with a limited mind and body.

Shukra - a general term for all male and female reproductive fluids, and for the hormones which cause them to be secreted.

Surya Namaskara - the Sun Salute, a series of Yogic exercises centering on the sun which strengthen and stabilize both mind and body.

Tamas - the cosmic force of inertia. Excess Tamas causes the mind to become dull and resistant to growth.

Tantra - from the root Tan, "to weave," Tantra weaves unformed energies into form. Traditionally Tantra refers to those practices which employ concentrated and refined energy for spiritual progress.

Tarpana - derived from the same root as the word Trpti, "satiation," Tarpana is an ancient method of disentangling one's consciousness from the obstructions created by one's genetic prakruti by satiating the personality created by those genes.

Tejas - the essence of cosmic Fire, which controls the mind's digestion and is transmitted via Ojas into the body's digestive system.

Triphala - "Three Fruits," a purifying and rejuvenating compound which is composed of Amalaki, Haritaki, and Bibhitaki, usually in equal proportions.

Tulsi - *Ocimum sanctum*, or holy basil, a variety of basil which is regarded as sacred and is used as medicine in fever, cancer, and many other conditions.

Upanishads - a group of explanations of the purport of the Vedas delivered by Rishis to their disciples.

Vedas - the ancient holy books of the Aryans, the oldest extant literary compositions of the human race.

Vipaka - the effect a substance has on an organism after it has been digested and assimilated into the system.

Virya - the "energy" of a food, medicine or poison; the enhancing or depressing effect a substance has on an individual organism's digestive power.

Vyadhikshamatva - literally "forgiveness of disease," by extension it refers to an organism's immunity, which depends on its ability to shrug off physical and mental insults.

Yoga - from the root Yuj, "to join," Yoga means joining or union. Traditionally Yoga is used as a general term for the disciplines which join the individual soul to the universal soul or cosmic consciousness.

Yukti - the process of creation of a specific effect by causing a number of essential factors to come together at the right place and time; it is derived from the root Yuj and is described as "generated from the union of many causes."

Index